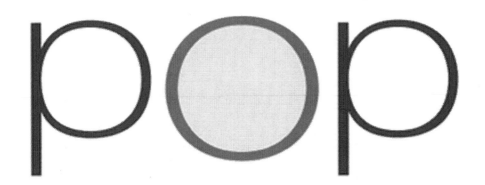

pop

BURST
THE DIET
BUBBLE

AND FINALLY LOSE WEIGHT

REBECCA CIPRIANO, MD
MS in Clinical Nutrition

with Kenneth Herman, EdD

To my husband, Joseph, and my daughter, Colette.
I love you both very much.

DISCLAIMER

The information contained in this book is based on the research and the personal and professional experiences of the authors. It is not intended as a substitute for consulting with a health care professional. The publisher and authors are not responsible for any adverse effects or consequences resulting from the use of any of the suggestions in this book. All matters pertaining to your physical and mental health should be supervised by a health care professional. The names of Dr. Cipriano's and Dr. Herman's patients described in this book and other identifying material have been changed. Any similarities to persons living or dead are coincidental.

WHAT EXPERTS SAY ABOUT *POP*

"This is a great book for anyone who wants to know not just how to lose weight but lose it for good by learning how to push past the mental block he or she has when it comes to achieving and then maintaining weight loss. Not your average weight loss how-to, this book actually gives readers guidelines for combating chronic conditions and mastering the lifestyle changes they need to lead a truly healthy life. By examining, understanding, and treating the person as a whole, Dr. Rebecca, complete with her unique brand of infectious motivation, is able to inspire a high level of lasting transformation from her patients.

"The book, divided into four main sections, gives readers an insight into the mind-set and processes of how to effectively achieve their own personal goals. 'Prescribing' specific everyday foods loaded with powerful nutrients, vitamins, and minerals along with a tried-and-tested fitness protocol and a few other handy weight loss tools, Dr. Rebecca shows how you can boost your ability to drop those excess pounds, get fit, prevent illness, reverse the effects of aging, and maintain optimal health.

"No one needs to be convinced that losing weight and getting healthy is the best way to go. What they do need is motivation and internal drive to actually do it, no matter what obstacles they face — and *Pop* does just that."

— **Neeti Misra, MD, FACOG**

"I have personally witnessed Dr. Rebecca Cipriano's weight loss program change the lives of many, many patients and friends. It is remarkable to see how well people respond to the program and how quickly they not just lose weight but are able to be free of medications for life-threatening conditions like diabetes and hypertension. It's also been amazing to see many of my patients who were once not able to conceive do the program and get pregnant naturally.

"The program works because it's a lifestyle change — one that's easy to follow with immediate and lasting results."

—Susan Pacana, MD, FACOG

"As a pediatrician, I've known Dr. Rebecca professionally for many years as an impressive OB/GYN physician with a large, thriving practice. Recently, I've known Dr. Rebecca personally as my weight loss mentor and coach, along with her team of nutritionists. Four years after I lost my husband to cancer, I had gained a lot of weight — on top of already being 20 pounds overweight. Dr. Rebecca was able to communicate with me at a professional and personal level, addressing my needs, and was always there when I needed her. I admire that when Dr. Rebecca is working with her weight loss patients (some of whom are teenagers from my practice), she not only offers personalized options based on each patient's needs but also takes the time to ensure her guidance is understood, well received, and capable of being applied with enthusiasm. Although I knew some weight loss–related information, it was Dr. Rebecca's knack for transmitting the knowledge in a way that spoke to me and inspired me to act on what I was learning. She empowered me to be accountable to myself and taught me how to create and keep good habits that brought about quick and massive changes in my life. For the first time in my struggle with weight loss, I lost 55 pounds and have kept 50 off for more than a year and counting.

"With her book, Dr. Rebecca is a trusted storyteller who empathetically educates by example. She understands the connection between one's emotional and physical needs and prescribes a weight loss solution based on each patient's personal situation and circumstances.

"I recommend Dr. Rebecca's book for men, women, and teens. As a matter of fact, I believe it is a guide to wellness for all."

—Zubaida Sadik, MD, FAAP

TABLE OF CONTENTS

PREFACE

Some of my nicest memories of childhood are eating fruit after dinner with my family, talking and laughing. My paternal grandfather had a wholesale fruit and vegetable business and my dad was always teaching us about how to pick the ripe fruit in season at the store. My parents encouraged healthy eating and junk food was a rarity.

I grew up and attended college in Maine and medical school in Chicago. The seed to become a doctor was planted when my maternal grandmother, Sarah — who in 1929 became the third woman to graduate from Northeastern Law School — suffered a stroke and came to live with us when I was 12. Caretaking tasks like helping her bathe and dress came naturally to me, unlike my squeamish older sister Debbie.

One day, while driving on Route 208 in Fair Lawn, New Jersey, sitting at a light outside the Nabisco factory, my father turned to me. "Boots," he said, using his nickname for me, "you are terrific with your grandmother and smart and caring — why don't you become a doctor?" And just like that, my career path was chosen.

In medical school, I was shocked that only one course in nutrition was introduced. That class was largely related to the treatment of nutritional deficiencies and didn't contain the nutrition education and connection with food and health that I had been hoping for. When my school offered a concordant master's degree in clinical nutrition, I jumped at the chance and completed my studies to graduate with a dual degree.

I decided to do my residency in obstetrics and gynecology, a field in which I still practice. However, the grueling hours, litigious nature of society these days, and fast pace of only having about 10 minutes to see each patient were not what I had intended for myself or my patients. Medicine the way it has evolved in the United States today is incredibly difficult. I began to feel more like a mouse on a wheel than a healer.

Enter the birth of my beautiful daughter, Colette. Also enter the 50 pounds I gained with her that I was having trouble shedding, and for a brief moment, I convinced myself that once you have a baby, you are just overweight and that is a law of nature.

Then I started really analyzing what I learned in my studies. Having the knowledge of what to do to be healthy was not enough until I put my knowledge into action and developed an organized plan — and so my weight loss program was born.

Many of my OB/GYN patients have medical problems that are related to their weight, which can affect them throughout all stages of life. I see a number of teenagers with irregular menstrual cycles. With extra weight, the estrogen/progesterone hormonal balance can be disrupted, and symptoms like worsening acne and hair growth can emerge. Continuing through a woman's life cycle, extra weight can lead to infertility through anovulation. Once a woman is pregnant, being overweight can lead to hypertension, diabetes, increased risk for cesarean section, and even increased risk of stillbirth. The list goes on and on. As menopause approaches, those patients not at a healthy weight are at an increased risk for uterine, ovarian, breast, and other cancers.

I began talking very seriously to all my patients about diet and exercise and quickly learned that I didn't have the time necessary to spend with them to really make a difference. It was then that my "aha!" moment came. I had the unique training to see the larger picture of weight loss and the obesity epidemic that faces our nation, and I knew that I could make an impact if given the right venue.

That led me to start a weight loss center in 2008, which has helped people lose more than 37,000 pounds at the time of this writing. Here's what some of those success stories say about the program:

"I wanted to thank you for helping me transform myself over the past six weeks. Hard to believe I lost 24 pounds and 5 inches so quickly. I didn't feel like your weight loss and exercise program was difficult to implement. It helped that you kept me focused and motivated. I feel more energetic, confident, and healthy. Going forward, I feel certain I can maintain my weight by continuing with your exercise program and using the knowledge you've given me on how to make the right food choices."

—Michael

"Over the past nine years, I have tried many programs, but Pop Weight Loss is by far the best one I've been on. I was able to stick to the program and feel satisfied. … I've lost 23 pounds and feel fabulous!"

—Marika

"The program is a complete and total lifestyle paradigm shift, but it's the easiest one you'll ever make. Smart food choices, working out, drinking water, and on-the-money coaching equal success. After the second week, I realized that I could do it. In fact, I never backslid. This is the program to do. The team at Dr. Rebecca's center is going to make sure that you lose the weight. My life is no different than yours. It's just as up and just as down. It's just as stressed out, over-scheduled, and underpaid. If the women of Pop Weight Loss can help me do it, then they can help you do it."

—Jillian

"Over the past 10 years, I have tried numerous weight loss plans and would lose weight but then gain back all I had lost and more. After my first session, I realized how bad my eating habits and food choices actually were. It was a relief to be able to just follow a healthy eating and exercise program. I have lost 50 pounds and have gone down four clothing sizes."

—Maureen

"I have kept my weight off for almost a year now. The team at Pop Weight Loss has helped me to maintain my weight by continuously altering my eating and exercise program to suit my busy lifestyle, has helped me keep my goals realistic, and has taught me the skills of self-discipline to make wise and healthy choices that will benefit my overall well-being and make me accountable to myself."

—Maryse

Whether you have five pounds or 205 pounds to lose, this book is written for you. It's also aimed at those who have lost weight in the past but been unsuccessful in keeping it off. More specifically, it is for all people who want to get healthy and really make a lifestyle change. If you follow the steps in this book, your life will be improved in many ways. Not only will you lose weight, but you'll have more energy and feel better about yourself.

I'll show you through my journey and some of my patients' journeys how you can accomplish your weight loss goals and feel years younger and sexier. Then I'll take you step by step through how to make a program that works for you. Recipes, sample menus, and a journal will help you stay on track. The reason this program is different from the rest — and the reason I've had such great success with it in the long term — is because this is a program with real food that you will be able to follow whether you are eating out or in.

Because weight loss isn't just a physical struggle but a mental one, my psychologist father, Dr. Kenneth Herman — yes, the very man who directed me toward medicine — has written a guide to how to avoid the mental pitfalls and be truly successful in your journey to get healthier. His comments stem from 50 years of experience in his field, during which time he's realized that there's a relationship between self-confidence and finding solutions to weight control and other life problems. He believes that a good body image and a positive outlook enhance self-esteem and are the catalysts to weight loss and living a life you are proud of. His advice on getting your mind in the right place in order to reach your goals is invaluable.

Diets do not work, but lifestyle changes do. I want you to take a journey with us to drop the idea of being on or off a "diet." You cannot constantly judge yourself by being good or being bad. This is where the concept of bursting the diet bubble stems from. This isn't a diet but a road to wellness. It's also not a race. Once you allow yourself to move forward and not judge yourself or your behavior, you will see that everyone stumbles, but if you keep moving in the right direction, the direction of health, you will win.

The book opens in Section 1 with case studies from weight loss patients with very commonly seen problems. Next, in Section

2, my psychologist father will help get you in the crucial mind-set for success through telling various patient stories, and he establishes why this is the time change will happen. Section 3 will be your chance to plug yourself into my easy formula and create your own personalized program. Last, the food guide in Section 4 gives you a large number of ideas on what to eat on your path to getting healthier.

I believe that I can help everyone who really wants to lose weight and feel better if they follow this program. There are many diet plans available, but there aren't many that give you the structure and psychological ammunition to succeed that this one does. The case histories of a medical doctor with an advanced degree in nutrition and those of a psychologist who has improved the lives of thousands will point you toward success with a multifaceted approach. Anyone can do this — all you need to do is follow the steps and you, too, will be leading a healthy life at the weight you want to be.

INTRODUCTION

The Three Pillars of Pop

We all waste energy on the small details of life. If you let these be a nuisance, you will not move forward with your goals. Weight loss is no different. Too many patients see weight loss as an insurmountable problem. The way weight loss is attacked in this book is with a step-wise, methodical approach in which you will be successful if you follow the program. What it's not is a strict diet that requires excluding major food groups or doing anything that harms your body.

Getting healthy isn't an overnight process, but it's also not complicated. The typical American dieter now makes four weight loss attempts per year, according to the U.S. Weight Loss & Diet Control Market study, with those attempts ringing up to $60.9 billion in 2010. If you're ready to burst that diet bubble and do something that's really effective, this is the plan for you. In my work, I've learned that for long-term weight loss, the following three components are essential: food, schedule, and exercise. It may seem simple, but these three crucial elements taken together make all the difference in the world. Teaching patients about them has become the backbone of our program.

1. FOOD

The food that you eat is so important — I can't overstate this enough. I don't believe in counting calories, weighing or measuring food, or prepackaged food. You cannot sustain the idea of constantly being on a "diet." It is imperative to think of your journey as a lifestyle change.

Countless patients come to me who have lost weight with shakes and bars or prepackaged systems like Jenny Craig and Nutrisystem, only to gain the weight back and more. The problem was that they could not make the transition back to real food, and more importantly, they never learned any nutritional information to make good choices. These, in my opinion, are temporary fad diets or quick fixes.

There is a serious crisis in our country and worldwide with chronic illnesses and obesity (which costs more than $190 billion a year in the U.S., according to the Institute of Medicine). The Centers for Disease Control and Prevention claims that 68.8 percent of the American population and up to 40 percent of our children are overweight or obese. Across the globe, 1 billion adults are overweight and 300 million are obese, says the World Health Organization. The scary news is that this is potentially only the beginning. By the year 2030 — if the current trend continues — an estimated 42 percent of adults in this country will be obese, and the number of people who are severely obese will double, says a recent study published in the *American Journal of Preventive Medicine*.

Obesity is known to be associated with increased risks of hypertension, diabetes, and cancer. According to Dr. Andrew Kagan in his book *Type 2 Diabetes*, type 2 diabetes affects close to 250 million people worldwide, including 27 million Americans. An estimated 79 million Americans are pre-diabetic and don't know it. Every year, more than a half million people die because of heart-related causes. You would think this alarming information would result in people taking better care of themselves; however, the number of illnesses related to the heart has not abated. The seven major heart disease risk factors are high cholesterol, increased blood pressure, high glucose levels, a sedentary lifestyle, smoking, an unhealthy diet, and being overweight.

These illnesses are largely a creation of too many processed foods, unhealthy fats, and sugars. On the whole, there is poor nutrition education in our schools and so much misinformation about food through advertising and the media that a lot of people are confused about what is healthy and what is not. I love teaching people to search mostly the periphery of the grocery store for fresh fruits and vegetables, lean proteins, fish, and whole grains (in moderation). I encourage incorporating fruits, vegetables, nuts, beans, and fish into their day to broaden the spectrum of food that they're eating. Healthy foods, especially fruits and vegetables, nuts, and beans, can prevent and even reverse diabetes, hypertension, and heart disease — that's a message that too few understand.

I want to stress that losing weight *will* reverse most medical problems, as this is a concept that helped me personally achieve my weight loss goal. We have to focus on food choices for the health and benefit of our bodies and not just comfort and pleasure. The medical community does not stress this and does not have the nutritional knowledge, the capacity, nor the time to discuss it with patients. The current medical climate is changing on a daily basis and putting more and more stresses and regulations on doctors, who now spend too much of their time treating chronic lifestyle diseases and not much time at all preventing them. Traditional medicine tells patients to lose weight but does not give them a clue as to how to actually do it.

While many individual doctors talk about the relationship between food and the impact it can have on reversing the disease process, the medical community as a whole, despite many advances, is slow to focus on this connection.

2. SCHEDULE

When I began devoting extended time to my patients and hearing about their days in relation to their eating habits, I sometimes wanted to fall off my chair. The amount of missed meals and meals on the go they mentioned was astonishing. I once had a patient tell me she installed a special tray (not unlike an airplane food tray) in her car so she could comfortably eat three meals. About 95 percent of my patients use the phrases "varies" or "all throughout the day" when asked the times of their meals. When you eat may seem like less of a problem than what you eat, but I believe they hold equal importance.

I work hard with my patients to establish a schedule of eating. I always need to adapt this to their life and schedule, whatever that may be. This can be tricky if someone needs to wake at 4 a.m. to be at a job by 6 a.m., or if the person works nights. But whether or not a person is working, has children, is a student, or has seven part-time jobs, the principles of eating on a schedule are the same and can be achieved even in a busy life.

In the beginning, I try to establish three meals and two snacks. I insist that the first meal be eaten within an hour to an hour and a half upon waking. Most overweight people skip breakfast. It is my belief that if you skip a meal, you make it up later because by the next time you eat, you are so hungry that you pick the wrong food, eat too fast, and have portions that are too large.

I also establish with patients the idea that it is snack time or mealtime *or it's not*! Far too many people graze or eat continuously throughout the day. This is not as bad if you are at a healthy weight but can be detrimental if you are overweight or obese. I ask patients to hear my words and say them to themselves — it's snack time or mealtime or it's not. This means that you are only involved with your food at your times of eating. You may skip a snack if you are truly not hungry, but no skipping any meals. I advise having dinner finished by 7 p.m. if possible and no snacking after dinner. When you eat late at night, you are often not hungry in the morning, and the poor pattern is perpetuated.

Americans do not eat in conjunction with their internal cues of being hungry or full — instead, a large study published in 2007 in the journal *Obesity* showed that Americans stop eating based on external cues. This means they do not stop when they are full, but they stop when the television show or sporting event is over. We must re-establish the internal hunger cue and learn to eat only when we are truly hungry.

Emotional eating is another big problem. My wonderful father, who is now 85 years old and holds a doctorate in psychology, addresses that in the second section of this book. The emotional component of weight loss can never be underestimated, and it is our belief that when you are at a positive place emotionally, you will be successful. Too many people eat when they are happy, when they are sad, and when they are stressed, tired, or bored. If, let's say, you are overeating because you are mad at your employer, then you are creating two problems: trouble at work and extra pounds. You must confront your problems directly and not eat as a result of them. His section of the book tackles how to overcome overeating obstacles, including:

- Emotional eating
- Triggers that make you want to eat when you're not hungry
- Thoughts, feelings, and emotional baggage from the past that keep you locked into poor eating habits
- Psychological barriers to exercise

- Turning off the negative "tapes" in your mind that say "I can't succeed … I've tried in the past and failed miserably; why should this be any different?"

My father teaches that you keep moving forward with your goals. Everyone has stumbling blocks along the way, but you can always pick yourself up and move on. No one can change your life but you. Believe these words and move forward — and keep that forward momentum even if you stumble a bit.

I try to help my patients slow down at mealtimes. We all run around too much during the day and do not make enough time for our meals. It takes your brain about 20 minutes to recognize that you have eaten. I have a Dr. Rebecca 18-minute rule I tell patients about. I tell them to check their watch and give themselves at least 18 minutes at mealtime to see if they are full. It is important to take time to chew your food well, plus it's better for digestion. I personally enjoy my food more when I can really taste the flavors. Additionally, try putting your fork down in between bites. Unconscious or mindless eating must be replaced by mindful eating. If after 18 minutes you are still hungry, have more food. I will bet that nine times out of 10, you'll be satiated.

In her book *Japanese Women Don't Get Old or Fat*, Naomi Moriyama describes *Hara hachi bunme*. This is a Japanese teaching that says to eat until you are 80 percent full because it allows your brain to keep pace with your stomach. I think this is brilliant, because Americans often eat too much and over-stretch their stomachs. The Japanese also do not fill the bowl or plate to the top. They have the lowest obesity rate in the world and have for the most part a wonderful diet of fresh fruits and vegetables, lots of soy, green tea, and fish filled with important omega-3 fatty acids.

3. EXERCISE

My third prong of the program, and one that completes a lifestyle change, is the exercise habit. I ask my patients to find the time and make it happen. For exercise, I have heard more excuses than I could have ever imagined. This needs to become a nonnegotiable habit just like brushing your teeth! It needs to become something that's automatic. Once you uncover a time that works and something you at least like to do, it becomes your sacred time. You must fit it into your day.

There is no doubt in my mind that exercise is crucial for the long-term maintenance of weight loss. Most of us push ourselves hard to work long hours and make money but do not push our bodies physically, nor do we know how to slow down and relax. We also have so many luxuries like cars and other conveniences that make it easy for us not to move much at all. Society was healthier hundreds of years ago when we needed to gather our own food and walk to destinations. I stress the importance of exercise by seeing this time not as a chore but as a break in the day that will help you focus, be more successful, and eventually keep the pounds off for good. It will be well worth the 30 minutes spent and give you the best chance of keeping weight off long term. My patients who hit their goal and stay at their goal weight become fanatical about continuing the exercise habit.

That's what's worked for me as well. I'm a busy doctor and mom who splits her time between personal commitments and working in the fields of weight loss and obstetrics/gynecology. I get up at 5 a.m. and run three to four miles every day, nonnegotiable (although I do walk if I feel tired). I have breakfast with my daughter by 6:30 a.m. and am on time for a 7:30 cesarean section at the hospital or an appointment in my office. I am no superwoman, but I stick to my schedule and make exercise a priority. I help people find their time, usually only 30 minutes a day, to do something they like and make it a part of their schedule. First, I think there is something magical about 30 minutes. Most people do not find it overwhelming. I also try to get people to see this time as their personal meditation time. Once they embrace that, I often get hugs from my patients of all ages for helping them bring exercise into their lives.

It is imperative to give exercise the same importance as your family or job or anything else that matters to you. Make it a priority! Exercise seems to be the great equalizer. Everyone who walks through my doors and follows my program loses weight, but those who keep it off maintain the exercise habit. This is well documented in the literature. A study in *Medicine and Science in Sports and Exercise* showed that people who maintained activity levels over 200 minutes per week (averaging 28 minutes a day) had improved health and the most successful maintenance of weight loss. If you can maintain a habit of regular exercise and eat properly, you are unlikely to ever have a weight problem again. It always baffles me when I sit with patients and tell them that this is the key to keeping the weight off, yet they still find excuses. Making excuses will never get you the results you want; it will only make you feel like a failure. You must change your thinking. This concept is so simple. It's time to grab it like a new religion and not make it more complicated than it is. Invariably, patients tell me that when they were happy with their weight, they were exercising regularly. This is not a coincidence; you must learn to combine exercise with good food choices. It is very difficult to maintain a healthy weight without both components.

If you have a lot of weight to lose, you may be slower to start with the exercise component. This is not uncommon and will come in time. The important point is staying on the path toward health. It is okay to start slowly and not push yourself beyond your comfort level at the beginning.

With these easy principles of food, schedule, and exercise, I have been so pleased with the fantastic results we achieve with my program. In just over four years, we have helped patients lose more than 37,000 pounds and live healthier lives. All of these components added together produce results. This formula works. What may vary is your commitment to grab it all at once. For me, the pace of losing weight is not important. If you want results quickly, I suggest you follow the plan diligently. If you need to ease into the process, that is okay, too. I hope you can identify with some aspects of my patients' case studies that will follow. Then we will provide you with a psychologist's guide to overcoming mental obstacles to make these changes permanent, and a step-by-step section on how to apply these principles to your own life, complete with food ideas.

It is this personal approach that has demystified weight loss for many others, and now it is your turn to experience the rewards of reaching your goal. We are thrilled to be with you on this wonderful journey toward improved health.

SECTION ONE

EAT PLAN MIND **BODY**

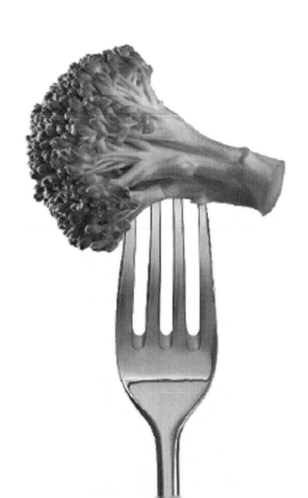

Many different life scenarios bring patients through my doors. It's interesting to see what makes someone ready or receptive to change. Usually they hit some sort of low point. Personally, I remember being about a year postpartum and needing to wear something other than maternity clothes to work. I went shopping and bought a new suit in a size 14 petite. Because I had a closet full of size 2 clothes, this was more than depressing for me. I also had to pay more than the suit cost to get it altered. When you are the weight you want to be, clothes fit much better. Shopping is fun instead of awful. I am always surprised at the tears that fall on many of my first encounters with patients. Somehow they get to a point where they know they need help and feel out of control with eating and disgusted with themselves.

While this is often related to clothing size for women, there are a whole host of other issues or events that lead people to change. The most common reason people seek help with weight loss is the onset of a new medical problem. Diabetes and hypertension are specifically linked with weight gain. Although it may sound strange, I love seeing these two problems because they are largely reversible when weight is lost — and watching those ailments fall away and not needing to be treated with medication is a huge motivator for people.

Other common life situations that inspire people to visit us at Pop Weight Loss are having a child, going through menopause, or becoming recently single. Sometimes a wedding or an upcoming life event can be motivating. Other times patients sustain an injury and are immobile for some time period in which they gain weight and are unable to lose it. Many times a picture from an important life event that shows excess weight triggers a change. This happened with my own husband, whom you will meet later in one of the case studies.

Regardless of the reason to seek help, the more upset a patient feels about his or her current weight or health situation, the more motivated that patient is to change. In this section, read seven real case studies from Pop Weight Loss — you just may find a situation that rings true for you. There are also tips along the way, drawn from the cases, to help anyone seeking to become healthier and happier.

CHAPTER 1

MARISOL, NEW-ONSET DIABETES

Age: 31
Height: 5'1"
Weight Pre-Pop: 190 pounds
Current Weight: 138 pounds
Occupation: Retail clothing store manager
Relationship Status: Newly married; no children

Marisol came to me for weight loss because her doctor told her that she would be on insulin injections for the rest of her life if she did not lose weight. She was only 31 years old at the time, worked full time, and wanted to get pregnant soon. I was thrilled that she came to me before pregnancy because I knew I could help her and that we would encounter fewer issues getting pregnant and during a pregnancy. Diabetes in pregnancy can lead to miscarriages, birth defects, higher incidence of cesarean section, and a whole host of other serious problems.

Marisol was smart to come and see me, as a diabetes diagnosis is not to be taken lightly. Type 2 diabetes has reached epidemic proportions, afflicting close to 250 million people worldwide — approximately 27 million in the United States alone — according to the book *Type 2 Diabetes* by Andrew Kagan, MD. This condition can lead to heart disease, stroke, kidney failure, amputation, and early death. The Centers for Disease Control and Prevention says that 33 percent of our children will eventually develop type 2 diabetes. But unlike type 1 diabetes, which appears as a genetic defect early in one's life, type 2 diabetes presents slowly and often is not detected until a crisis occurs. The good news is that even though some people do have a genetic potential to develop type 2 diabetes, with attention to diet and eliminating processed foods and sugars, type 2 diabetes is reversible.

Marisol had problems with all three of my mainstay Pop Weight Loss areas (food, schedule, and exercise), but one stood out more than the others and seemed to be the core of her struggles. While Marisol's schedule was off a bit and she had no real exercise plan, her main problem could be summed up in one word: *tortilla.* She was eating tortillas for breakfast, lunch, and dinner! I remember a session when Marisol was crying real tears hearing the news that her beloved corn tortillas were a huge factor in her becoming diabetic at such a young age. "Tortillas are love," she said as she cried. "Marisol, your family is love — not tortillas," I told her. We laugh about it now.

PRESCRIPTION

I had to get Marisol off the tortilla trail and onto a healthier lifestyle path. Corn, the main ingredient in Marisol's tortillas, is very high on the glycemic index and can raise blood sugars quickly. This was the exact opposite of what we wanted for Marisol. Also, when patients have a particular trigger food, whether it's chocolate or tortillas, my advice is almost always to *stay away*. Trigger foods are just that — triggers — and usually we cannot control the amount consumed at all. I created a new schedule of eating for Marisol that involved three meals and two snacks. For her, the emphasis was on combining a protein (or a better carbohydrate source that included 100 percent whole wheat or whole grain) with a fruit or a vegetable for every meal and every snack. I also got her focusing on vegetables and beans as her main foods instead of tortillas so we could bring antioxidants and nutrient-rich foods into her day.

Here's a sample day in food choices for Marisol:

Breakfast: egg whites with spinach, mushrooms, and tomato or oatmeal with berries

Mid-morning snack: apple and natural peanut butter

Lunch: salad with fish or beans and soup/salad

Mid-afternoon snack: veggies and hummus

Dinner: wild salmon, lentils, and broccoli with fresh cantaloupe for dessert

We eliminated her nighttime snacking altogether. We also worked hard to carve out time in her day for exercise. Marisol had the common misconception that because she was active during the day, it counted as exercise. She worked long hours and complained that she was not a morning person. It was during a weekly session that Marisol realized she was still not making the time to exercise. She agreed to change to morning exercise. After working with thousands of patients, I know that the morning is the preferred time. Life happens and too many other things get in the way. I also think that people should be able to have their evenings to relax and not have the added pressure of exercise. I asked her for one half hour of any cardiovascular exercise seven days a week. She chose to walk and also started to get to bed earlier — a crucial change, as we need about seven hours of sleep for successful weight loss.

Outcome

Marisol lost 52 pounds in seven months and reached her goal weight — a weight she had not been since age 18. She is not diabetic and has become a morning exercise person. She also enjoys her beloved tortillas two to three times a week. She has learned that she can have them the way her mom taught her to make them, but not every day and not four times a day. Marisol recently told our staff she is pregnant. We are so happy for her and I know her pregnancy and life will be easier and healthier without diabetes.

Diabetes Warning Signs

If you have any of the following symptoms, talk to your doctor about whether you should be screened for diabetes:

- Increased thirst
- Increased, extreme hunger
- Dry mouth
- Frequent urination or urine infections
- Unexplained weight loss
- Fatigue and irritability
- Blurred vision
- Cuts and bruises that are especially slow to heal
- Tingling or numbness in your hands or feet

CHAPTER 2

ISAAC, NEW-ONSET HYPERTENSION AND KNEE PAIN

Age: 53
Height: 5'8"
Weight Pre-Pop: 225 pounds
Current Weight: 161 pounds
Occupation: Investment banker
Relationship Status: Married; one daughter

Isaac came to me because he had just been prescribed high blood pressure medicine and did not want to take it. He also had chronic fatigue and complained about knee pain. At our first consultation, it was clear to me that while food choices and lack of exercise were indeed a problem for Isaac, his schedule of eating and sleeping was his true downfall. The first time I met Isaac, his eyes were tired and the buttons on his crisp white shirt were popping.

Isaac had to get up at 3:30 a.m. in order to be in his office in New York City at 7 a.m. Because he was regularly getting home past 7 p.m., he stayed up to be with his family and often went to bed at midnight. Isaac was functioning on only three and a half hours of sleep. Impossible.

PRESCRIPTION

I had to completely revamp Isaac's schedule. He needed to get to bed by 9 so he could have at least six and a half hours of sleep. He talked with his family about his need to sleep more, and of course they were supportive. I also had him eat something before he left his house at 4 a.m. Getting him to eat within an hour of waking and then have a snack around 8 a.m. made a huge difference in his life. Previously, he was eating for the first time around 9 a.m. and usually it was a bagel or muffin. Getting up at 3:30 a.m. and not eating until 9 a.m. meant going five and a half hours without food, which was causing Isaac to binge later in the day. His food choices needed help, too. While bagels and muffins are comforting, both have very little protein and very little nutritional value. Isaac also traveled frequently and had many meals in restaurants. We taught him better food choices, whether eating out or at home. Learning to make good choices wherever you are is a big part of mindful eating and a large component of Pop Weight Loss. Restrictive diets do not work. Once you learn how to order properly, it is possible to eat out regularly, lose weight, and maintain it. This can truly be done in any diner or five-star restaurant.

Here's a sample day in food for Isaac:

4 a.m.: Greek yogurt and berries

8 a.m.: egg whites with vegetables

Noon: grilled chicken salad or soup with salad

3 p.m.: vegetables with guacamole or bean dip

7 p.m.: grilled scallops, green beans, a sweet potato, and red grapes

We also started an exercise regimen and Isaac was able to take advantage of the gym at his company.

Hypertension and weight gain are closely linked. A normal blood pressure is 120/80. A blood pressure of 140/90 and above is considered high. The higher your blood pressure, the more potential damage to your arteries and the higher your risk of a heart attack or stroke. I've had patients as young as 29 years old who have had heart attacks and other related medical problems. The American Heart Association reports that a third of U.S. adults have hypertension and some don't know it. The good news is that a 2007 Italian study found that a modest decrease in weight of even 5 percent can decrease your blood pressure. This was true for Isaac.

OUTCOME

Isaac lost 64 pounds and never ended up needing blood pressure medication. Isaac's knee pain disappeared. Prior to coming to see me, he had been to an orthopedic surgeon who had told him his knees were fine but that he needed to lose weight. He didn't believe it until he proved it to himself. Isaac's wife also joined the program and reached her goal weight. They both still weigh in with us regularly and lead very healthy lives. Prior to coming to Pop Weight Loss, Isaac ate very little fish and felt his meal was not complete without beef or chicken. Now he eats fish or a vegetarian entree about four times a week and has learned to enjoy it, along with his new body.

Getting Better Sleep

Isaac was trying to operate on three and a half hours of sleep, which simply isn't enough. Most adults need between seven and eight hours a night, although some may need as little as five or as many as 10 hours. With an adequate amount of sleep, not only will you be able to function better during the day, but it'll also be easier to lose weight.

To get the best sleep possible, keep the following sleep hygiene tips in mind:

- Don't eat or drink close to bedtime.
- Try to go to sleep and wake up at the same time every day.
- Don't take your worries to bed.
- Avoid taking naps during the day if you can.
- Don't use your bed for watching TV, reading, or doing work.
- Make your bedroom cool and comfortable.
- Take a bath before you go to sleep. Adding Epsom salts is helpful.

CHAPTER 3

JEN, POSTPARTUM WEIGHT GAIN AND DEPRESSION

Age: 35
Height: 5'2"
Weight Pre-Pop: 170 pounds
Current Weight: 132 pounds
Occupation: Stay-at-home mom
Relationship Status: Married; two children

Jen is a very sweet mother of two boys, 1 and 3. On our first visit, Jen cried and told me she is completely out of control with eating. She said she did not have a weight problem until having children, and it was making her depressed. The month prior, her primary care doctor had prescribed an antidepressant. Since starting the medication, she felt her mood was slightly better, but now she felt numb emotionally. She had put on another 15 pounds in the six weeks since she started the medication.

Nights were a huge problem for Jen. Her husband worked late most nights and Jen found herself putting her children to bed and then binge eating. She convinced herself that she needed to eat to stay awake and talk with her husband, but she usually fell asleep before he came home. She also felt that the nights were her time to relax, yet the time was now primarily being spent eating. Jen worked in an office before her children were born, and she missed the stimulation at work, the interaction with her co-workers, and even getting dressed for work. She loved her children deeply but felt isolated and alone.

PRESCRIPTION

It is well documented that mood disorders and weight are closely linked. I would estimate that 70 percent of my weight loss patients have been clinically depressed at one time, and Jen showed some classic symptoms of depression. She suffered from anhedonia, a condition in which you don't enjoy the things you used to enjoy. Jen was lonely and overwhelmed in her new role as a mom, and her health and weight were suffering. She needed a lifestyle overhaul.

I encouraged Jen to join her local YMCA, which was a good choice for her for many reasons. First, I wanted to get her exercising and the YMCA had day care. I wanted to get Jen out of the house more, and I knew she would meet other new moms who were going through similar issues. When she first started exercising, she tried to go on the treadmill and the elliptical machine. She had trouble focusing and felt worried about her kids in day care. I encouraged Jen to take some classes and told her the caregivers would come and find her if they needed help with the boys. Zumba and spin classes were the ones that got Jen motivated the most. She made some friends and started to make plans for playdates outside the gym. She felt relieved that she was not the only mom struggling with her new role.

Jen's food was the next item on the list needing an overhaul. Jen felt tortured by her kitchen and the food there. I had her clean out the kitchen of the foods that haunted her and called her name. She confessed that most of the foods she overate were snack foods she had bought for the kids. We had to focus on only buying healthy foods, for both her and the kids, and clearly defining times for snack times and mealtimes. We also had to draw a line between Jen's food and her children's food. Many parents finish their kids' food because they don't want to waste it. We talked with Jen about wrapping up the unfinished food immediately. Mindlessly finishing it was not an option. By doing this, Jen discovered how good it felt to be hungry by mealtime instead of snacking throughout the day as she had done previously.

We replaced Jen's snacking with a protein plus a fruit or a vegetable for every snack and every meal. The old Jen would snack on pretzels and Goldfish crackers and feel hungry afterward. The new Jen enjoyed plain low-fat Greek yogurt with fresh fruit. Greek yogurt is a fantastic choice because it is low in sugar, high in protein, and acts as a probiotic for your intestinal track, which improves digestion and can relieve constipation. At 10 a.m. every morning, she and her older son would have an apple and peanut butter party. Jen was thrilled that she wasn't hungry and felt in control of her eating.

I also love the idea of moms sharing meals with their kids rather than acting as servants. Jen was wasting time making separate meals for her picky 3-year-old. Because kids' palates change so much, it's crucial for them to keep trying new foods. I see too many adults who have all sorts of crazy food hang-ups, and I blame mom and dad for not breaking these habits. I see adults who eat no fish, or nothing green, or no real vegetables. Kids must be given healthy choices when they are hungry, and they will eat.

Last but not least, we had to deal with the nighttime eating issue. We stuck to the rule of no eating after dinner and instituted some herbal tea time. Now instead of binge eating, Jen would enjoy her favorite television shows and catch up on home chores, and most nights she was awake when her husband came home. She started enjoying her quiet time and feeling good about herself again.

OUTCOME

Jen lost 38 pounds and found herself. She came off the antidepressant medication and has a healthy relationship with food. Jen talked with her husband and made plans to return to work part-time when her youngest is 2. Knowing that the time at home is not permanent helped Jen to slow down and enjoy this time more.

Note: If you are feeling depressed like Jen, I urge you to seek help. A good place to start is your family doctor.

Finding the Right Gym (or Exercise) for You

For Jen, the local YMCA was the best choice, given its child care option, chance to meet other moms in a similar situation, and exercise amenities provided. How do you know what the right gym is for you? Here are some points to take into consideration:

1. The convenience factor
At the end of the day, you're unlikely to be happy with your gym unless it's relatively convenient to get to — close to your house or workplace, with operating hours that fit your schedule. The farther away it is, the more excuses you'll make not to go.

2. The exercise options
Do you like taking classes? Are you mostly interested in the cardio equipment? Is swimming in a pool or having a yoga studio important? Look at what you like to do now, and what you'd like to do in the future — this is a place you'll be spending a lot of time, so there should be a variety of exercise options that excite you.

3. The price
Typically, the more amenities a gym has, the higher the membership cost. Find an option that works with your budget. This is an investment in your health, but with some fancy gyms, you may be paying for amenities you'll never use.

Also, don't forget that no gym membership is always an option. Some people prefer using a home gym, working out to DVDs, or walking outside. If you're not a gym person — or there's no good location for you — consider at-home alternatives. This is certainly a time-efficient choice.

CHAPTER 4

FRED, CHRONIC YO-YO DIETER

Age: 58
Height: 5'9"
Weight Pre-Pop: 250 pounds
Current Weight: 186 pounds
Occupation: Real estate broker
Relationship Status: Divorced; two grown children

W hen Fred first came to me, he sat in the consult with his arms folded tight. He told me he is divorced, does not have a refrigerator, and eats all meals at restaurants. He said he did not plan to change his routine. I told him I was okay with that but was secretly feeling sad that he would not enjoy any meals at home. He told me that he had gained and lost the same 50 pounds over and over again since he was 30. He'd been on every weight program under the sun with some success on all, but his current weight was the heaviest he had ever been. A recent physical exam with his internist resulted in adding cholesterol medicine to his prescription regimen, joining the hypertension medication he was already taking.

Fred's real problem was that he never completed a lifestyle change with all the programs he tried. He never learned good food choices and never developed a *habit* of exercise. "Every time I attained a weight that I was happy with, I was exercising," he said. "Then something happened like a vacation or a minor injury and I would stop exercising." He told me the last time he was happy with his weight, his gym went out of business and he never found a new one. Then the weight slowly returned and he was worse off than when he started.

I cannot tell you how common this theme is with yo-yo dieters. For me, a weight loss doctor, it is exhausting to hear people tell their stories because I can feel the pain they've been experiencing for decades. Luckily, there is a solution. For anyone who is a yo-yo dieter, developing a true habit of exercise protects and maintains any weight loss. Truly bursting the concept of being on or off a diet is crucial for success.

PRESCRIPTION

First, we needed to rework Fred's food choices. I asked him to bring in the menus from the restaurants he frequented. They numbered about 15. We concentrated on healthy choices to replace what he usually ate.

The breakfast changes were fairly easy. The basic principles of Pop Weight Loss came into action. For food, we started pulling out unhealthy fats and sugars. Fred's usual bacon and eggs, a bagel with cream cheese, or a blueberry muffin became oatmeal with fruit or egg whites with vegetables (with Canadian bacon once a week). Even though oatmeal and a bagel are both considered carbohydrates, they are worlds apart. Oatmeal (steel-cut or plain, not flavored) is a far better choice than the refined carbohydrates in a bagel or muffin. Bagel sizes have become enormous, and the calories in one bagel can exceed 600. The egg-white omelet with vegetables or plain oatmeal with fruit have more fiber and will keep you fuller longer. They also will not spike your blood sugar so high that you'll have a rapid drop about an hour later, leaving you dead tired and looking for something else to eat or drink to pick you up.

Fred's lunch changed from sandwiches to salads with protein or soup. Because Fred was largely a meat and potatoes guy, it was a challenge to get him to eat alternate proteins. This definitely did not happen overnight. He needed to change gradually and told us he could not live on bird food. I have two approaches to this type of resistance that usually are effective. First, I had Fred try using meat as a condiment. I had him start with chicken salad or steak salad either for lunch or dinner instead of a sandwich. This was important so he could get used to the idea of eating smaller amounts of meat. I'm always trying to move patients away from saturated fat in animal proteins and interest them in foods with monounsaturated fat — the good fat that lowers cholesterol — like nuts and beans. Fred did well having a Greek salad for lunch. He enjoyed the feta cheese and olives and found he was less tired in the afternoon than he had been before.

Next I asked Fred to consume fish for dinner once a week. He resisted. He told me he loved tomato sauce. I asked him to order sautéed or grilled mild fish like flounder and ask the restaurant to put tomato sauce on it. It was a miracle — he liked it. He was to try one more fish dish a week from then on. I have had a lot of success changing diets from mostly chicken and beef to nuts, beans, fish, and salads; although it can be difficult, it's such an important transition.

Soups were introduced at lunch for Fred, too. He liked lentil soup, escarole and beans, and even turkey or vegetarian chili.

The fiber, protein, and monounsaturated fat in beans, very much underutilized in American diets, have tremendous health benefits. A few months into the program, Fred said he was surprised that he was feeling so healthy. He told us that he would usually have at least three colds during the winter but was pleased that he had not gotten any this season. It was likely the antioxidants and phytochemicals that Fred was getting from his fruits, vegetables, nuts, and beans that were giving him immunity against many everyday illnesses. Knowing this helped Fred stay on track.

Fred's dinners were easy to fix. We asked Fred to forgo the bread basket and concentrate on protein plus vegetables as a template. If, for example, his grilled fish came with risotto, he would ask for sautéed vegetables instead. He had many business dinners where food and alcohol were served in abundance. We had started Fred on three fruits a day, and I usually advised one with breakfast, one with a morning snack, and the last one after dinner. If Fred wanted one drink with dinner, he would use that in place of one fruit for the day. I find it important to stick with the one-drink rule. After counseling thousands of people, I've realized that more than one drink is big trouble. Too often, excess alcohol leads to excess food and dessert intake. Also eliminated were any sweet drinks made with too much sugar (like margaritas). I didn't ask Fred to stop drinking completely, though — when you are on a lifestyle journey change, I don't think it's realistic to never have alcohol if you drink. Extremely restrictive diets are impossible to follow and are usually a recipe for failure.

Probably the hardest challenge we had with Fred was getting him to exercise regularly. He refused morning exercise, did not like to exercise anywhere but a gym, and kept blaming work as an excuse not to exercise. I told him if we found a time that worked, he would never yo-yo again. I talked with him about thinking of that time as meditation time, sacred time. We figured out that after work but before dinner was a reasonable time for him. He started going straight from work at 5:30 p.m. Once he began scheduling all other appointments before this time, things started to fall in place. This is an important point. Fred chose to schedule in his exercise time; he made it a priority. After work but before dinner is my second favorite exercise time behind first thing in the morning and seems to work for men in particular or with women who have to be at work early but are home from work at an earlier hour.

OUTCOME

It took Fred almost one year to hit his goal. He had many plateaus along the way. The exercise habit proved the most difficult for him, and it was not until he saw for himself that a good week included *regular* exercise that he hit his final goal, which was to lose 64 pounds. Fred still comes in to weigh in regularly and still does not own a refrigerator — even with that considerable challenge, he doesn't have to take the cholesterol medication the internist prescribed and brags that he never gets sick. Can you imagine the personal satisfaction he is getting? Fred is very proud of himself, and justifiably so.

Drink Responsibly

Fred learned to eliminate alcoholic drinks with too much sugar in them — like margaritas — but can still enjoy an adult beverage in moderation. Here's what to keep in mind if imbibing:

Limit your consumption to one glass of beer, wine, or hard alcohol per day, if at all. If you have a drink, have one fewer serving of fruit that day (usually people start this plan with three fruits a day). Look for the lowest total carbohydrate grams you can find. One good option is to combine half a glass of wine with seltzer to make a spritzer.

Here are some other decent choices:

BEER

Serving size: 12 ounces

Bud Light: 110 calories, 6.6 grams carbs
Budweiser Select: 99 calories, 3.1 grams carbs
Budweiser Select 55: 55 calories, 1.9 grams carbs
Busch Light: 95 calories, 3.2 grams carbs
Coors Light: 104 calories, 5.3 grams carbs
Corona Light: 105 calories, 5 grams carbs
Leinenkugel Light: 105 calories, 5.7 grams carbs
Leinenkugel Amber Light: 110 calories, 7.4 grams carbs
Michelob Ultra: 95 calories, 2.6 grams carbs
Miller Lite: 96 calories, 3.2 grams carbs
Miller Genuine Draft Light: 64 calories, 2.4 grams carbs
Milwaukee's Best Light: 98 calories, 3.5 grams carbs
Rolling Rock Green Light Low Carb Beer: 83 calories, 2.4 grams carbs
Thin Ice: 90 calories, 1 gram carbs

WINE/CHAMPAGNE

Serving size: 5 ounces and 5 grams carbs

Dry White (e.g., Sauvignon Blanc, Chardonnay): ~100 calories, ~3 grams carbs
Dry Red (e.g., Syrah, Pinot Noir, Cabernet Sauvignon): ~120-125 calories, ~3.5 to 4 grams carbs
Zinfandel: 130 calories, 4.2 grams carbs
Champagne (3.5 ounces): 87 calories, 5 grams carbs

HARD LIQUOR

Serving size: 1.5 ounces

Gin/Scotch/Whiskey/Rum: 56 calories, 0 grams carbs
Tequila: 60 calories, 0 grams carbs (and non-sedating)
Vodka: 56 calories, 0 grams carbs

SKINNYGIRL COCKTAILS

Serving size: 1.5 ounces

Cocktails: 35.5 calories, 1.8 grams carbs
Margaritas: 37.5 calories, 1.4 grams carbs
Avoid any drink mixes other than Skinnygirl because of the high sugar content.

CHAPTER 5

BRITTANY, TEENAGE OBESITY

Age: 16
Height: 5'5"
Weight Pre-Pop: 190 pounds
Current Weight: 138 pounds
Occupation: Student
Relationship Status: Single

Like many teens, Brittany came to me with a full schedule and poor eating habits. She often skipped breakfast, and because she is an excellent student, she stayed up late studying and found herself snacking on chips, cookies, and other junk foods. Gym class once a week was the only bit of exercise she was getting.

After a visit to her pediatrician, Brittany and her mom realized she needed help to lose weight. Her cholesterol was elevated and her fasting glucose was high. Even at her young age, she was headed toward diabetes and cholesterol medication. Brittany had tried Weight Watchers but was very frustrated that she had only lost two pounds in a month. Brittany's mom desperately wanted to help her daughter, but she didn't know how to.

I had an instant connection with Brittany. She is a lovely, vibrant teen who is witty and warm and aspires to be a medical doctor, specifically an oncologist. When we explored her past, I learned that Brittany has struggled most of her life with weight issues. Her genetic makeup is just like her father's: big-boned without delicate features. While her mom tried to cook healthy foods for her, Brittany's hectic schedule made her eating habits a major problem.

Brittany is not alone in her struggles. The Centers for Disease Control and Prevention reports that 17 percent, or 12.5 million, of children and adolescents age 2 to 19 are obese (when those who are overweight are added, the figure rises to 40 percent). Since 1980, the prevalence of obesity in children and adolescents has almost tripled.

PRESCRIPTION

Making good food choices and eating a better variety of foods were the first actions to be taken. Brittany's diet was full of blunders. She loved ketchup on everything and piled it on! We had a serious ketchup problem that added tons of sugar to her diet. Too much of any single food item is always problematic.

Because I knew Brittany was interested in fighting cancer, I started teaching her about the antioxidant and anti-inflammatory properties of certain fruits and vegetables. Antioxidants are chemicals found in fresh fruits and vegetables that fight free radicals, molecules that can cause cell damage and inflammation in our bodies. It is the antioxidants in fruits and vegetables that can fight and possibly prevent cancers. Tomatoes, for example, contain lycopene (found in most red fruits and vegetables), which can protect our skin from skin cancer, so I suggested that Brittany trade in the sugar-laden ketchup for a fresh tomato salsa or an unsweetened tomato sauce or paste instead. I also gave her permission to use reduced-sugar ketchup, which she told me tasted almost the same as the real stuff.

Going out with her friends and being selective regarding what she ate was hard for Brittany. We found that this just took a little extra planning on her part. When she was out at a pizza place, she knew she could order a grilled chicken salad or chef salad and still be just as happy enjoying time with her friends. Brittany also had a busy social calendar with lots of parties to attend. We had her eat a small meal prior to going so that she would not show up starved. She kept almonds in her purse so that if she found herself in a pizza-only situation, she would have something to snack on. She could then decide for herself if she would like one slice of pizza or if she would pass on it. It was a struggle to get Brittany to try different foods, especially fish and beans. Fortunately, her mom is supportive and just kept trying until we had a few she liked. Brittany now eats salmon, tilapia, and scallops, which are all new for her.

One of my biggest pieces of advice to Brittany was not to skip breakfast. This is a major issue for a lot of people, especially teenagers. Skipping breakfast sets up the day for failure. If you skip a meal, you end up making it up later and usually invite poor choices and overeating. I am also a big fan of recommending not eating after 7 p.m. for most people. This is a very good habit to get into and really helps most people sleep better and become hungry for breakfast the next morning. If Brittany felt hungry at night, we had a strict fruits-and-nuts-only rule. I do this with my own daughter, who gets hungry after dinner, and I think it works well.

Exercise was also a component that I am thrilled to say Brittany took to like a new religion. She and her mom had joined the gym in their town and went together regularly every afternoon. We specifically picked the afternoon so Brittany would be able to maintain the workout schedule as she transitioned from summer to the school year. It is vital to change your exercise and eating schedule when your actual schedule changes. She figured out herself that if her exercise was good that week, then the weight loss averaged three pounds a week. Once this happened, she was motivated to exercise without me telling her to. There was no stopping her because the new habits clicked.

OUTCOME

At the writing of this book, Brittany is going back to school 52 pounds lighter than she was last year. She is truly an inspiration. We need to work hard to get her to her goal, which is just 20 pounds away now. We also need to carefully transition her to her new school schedule. I am very proud of Brittany and love that she accepts the challenge when I push her. She's helped other teens in the program who are struggling, which warms my heart. Brittany is so focused and determined to succeed that I truly forget that she is just 16 years old — proof that you can change your life at any age.

4 Tips for Eating Out

If socializing in restaurants is part of your routine like it is for Brittany, here are four quick tips to keep the outings high on fun and low on poor food choices:

- Plan ahead. Look up the menu options beforehand. That way, you can go in with an idea of what you can order that will work with your weight loss goals. Having that set beforehand will help you resist an on-the-spot poor choice.
- Know what menu words to look for. If you see the following, it probably means the dish was prepared in a way that's not as healthy as you'd like: *fried, sautéed, creamed, buttered, braised, basted, pan-fried, au gratin,* and *scalloped.* Smarter choices are *baked, grilled, steamed,* and *poached.*
- Don't feel like you have to clear your plate. If the dish is too big (as it is in most American restaurants these days), you can share your meal with a friend, box up whatever's left over, or just leave some on the plate. Consider asking the waiter to box up half your meal before you begin so you won't be tempted to eat it all in one sitting.
- Get your dressing on the side. Salads are often a good choice, but once you add the dressing, they can quickly shift from low-cal to surprisingly high in fat. Put yourself in control of how much dressing you eat by getting it on the side and dipping your fork into it to pick up just a little of the flavor for each bite (don't pour it, or you'll defeat the purpose of getting it on the side).

CHAPTER 6

TRICIA, MORBID OBESITY AND UTERINE CANCER

Age: 39
Height: 5'8"
Weight Pre-Pop: 360 pounds
Current Weight: 253 pounds
Occupation: Full-time hospital administrative work in the oncology department
Relationship Status: Married; two children, 7 and 9

Tricia is one of the nicest people I know. She is warm and kind and always smiling. I delivered both her children. We've always shared a nice relationship and I was able to tell Tricia bluntly and directly when I was worried about her medical conditions and her weight. We had two relatively uneventful pregnancies and vaginal deliveries with gestational diabetes and hypertension that were manageable. This was fortunate considering her size. In the first few years of my weight loss program, I tried very hard to get Tricia to come in, but for some reason, she was not yet ready. It wasn't until a gynecology condition called atypical hyperplasia occurred that Tricia was able to tackle her very serious weight condition. She had finally realized that losing weight was a necessity.

The hormonal balance between estrogen and progesterone in women is what keeps a woman's menstrual cycle regular. Extra adipose, or fat, cells can lead to a disruption in the balance, causing heavy and irregular bleeding and sometimes even masculinizing side effects like acne, deepening of the voice, and excess hair. This happens because extra adipose can increase testosterone production. Tricia came to me with very heavy periods, and an endometrial (or uterine) biopsy done in the office showed complex endometrial hyperplasia with atypia — a condition that leads to uterine cancer in 30 percent of people who have it. The treatment for this condition is almost always a hysterectomy, but because Tricia's weight made her a poor surgical candidate, we chose to treat her with chemotherapy.

Shortly after this treatment, she walked into my Freehold, N.J., office and said, "Dr. Rebecca, I'm ready."

"Ready for what?" I asked.

"Your weight loss program," she replied. It wasn't until she had a scare with cancer that she was really ready to change. Unfortunately, it often takes a crisis to make people in need of help receptive to seeking it.

Tricia was morbidly obese with a BMI of 55. (See the sidebar at the end of this chapter for an explanation of BMI.) Her husband, Todd, who is truly supportive and whom I already knew from her pregnancies, came to the consult with her. He had tears in his eyes when I showed them where Tricia fell on the BMI scale. He said, "Please help us; we trust you." At this point, I had tears in my eyes.

PRESCRIPTION

Tricia had been heavy since age 2. Her parents were heavy, as were her grandparents. When most members of a family are overweight, creating new habits is most difficult. I think postpartum weight gain, menopause weight gain, and even smoking cessation weight gain are easier to manage. These situations are usually a few years in duration at most. Nothing is easy, and hard work is behind every success, but someone who has had a severe weight problem his or her entire life is my toughest patient. To her credit, Tricia worked diligently and never looked back.

First, we reworked her food choices. She was not making ideal choices, but they were not the worst, either. Tricia fell into a lot of food misconception traps. For example, the old Tricia was eating cereal in the morning and drinking orange juice. Most breakfast cereals are loaded with carbohydrates. Even those that claim health or have some whole-grain redeeming values, like Kashi GoLean, have too much sugar and not enough protein. They are not so different from the bad choices of bagels and muffins. I started Tricia on a high-protein, low-carbohydrate breakfast cereal (less than 15 grams total carbohydrates per cup) plus berries in the morning. The berries are a great source of antioxidants. I suggest most of my patients have at least 1 cup of berries each day. The orange juice had far too much sugar, so I asked Tricia to opt for fruit instead. The fiber and antioxidants in one orange are far superior to any sugar-laden cup of juice. When a goal weight is reached, small amounts of fruit juice can be enjoyed.

Tricia was also eating way too much. Remember the Dr. Rebecca 18-minute rule, in which your brain doesn't know you have eaten until at least 18 minutes have passed. Tricia's busy life of working full time, taking care of two kids, and rushing after work to get them to their sporting events and practices left her eating on the fly. When you don't have a minute to slow yourself down, you can get used to big portions very quickly. So we needed to do everything we could to bring a slower pace to Tricia's day. This started with getting to bed earlier. Remember, most of us need at least seven hours of sleep a night to achieve regular weight loss. Also, Tricia never really snacked. She left her house early to be at work by 8 and often didn't have lunch until after 1. This is too long to go between meals. She would feel so hungry by lunch that she would eat a sandwich and potato chips as quickly as she could. After this type of lunch, people often feel very tired and look for something after lunch to wake them up. Having regular snacks and not waiting until you are starved is a much smarter approach.

I started Tricia on a schedule that included:

Breakfast at 6:30 a.m.: high-protein cereal with berries, or egg whites with vegetables

Snack at 9:30 a.m.: almonds plus an apple or a pear

Lunch at noon: salad plus protein (more fish, less chicken) or bean soup

Snack at 3:30 p.m.: a raw vegetable plus protein like low-fat cheese or hummus

Dinner by 7 p.m.: lean protein plus a cooked vegetable and the last fruit of the day

Tricia could not believe that she didn't feel starved. She also had much more energy during the day. We continued the slow-yourself-down attitude at dinner. I asked Tricia to focus on one plate of food eaten *slowly* over at least 18 minutes. Previously, she used to place the food in the center of the table and continued to serve herself and the family because they were usually rushing somewhere. She liked this idea of having just one plate and putting her fork down between bites, drinking water, and leaving at least 18 minutes to eat and chew properly. Chewing your food well and savoring it is much better for digestion. Tricia also worked to eat more fish for dinner and came to the realization that prior to starting the program, she was eating a portion three times the size it should have been (one serving of fish should be the size of your hand) due to her habit of eating so quickly.

Tricia also dived right into the exercise habit, not missing a single day. She knew she didn't like to exercise alone, so she organized a neighborhood exercise class from 5 to 6 a.m. Getting others to join her in working out added to her motivation, and she felt proud to inspire her friends. She knew if her exercise time was not the first thing in the morning, she would not return to it after work.

OUTCOME

I am pleased to report that Tricia is down a whopping 107 pounds in about 10 months. That amazing drop in weight did not happen overnight, but Tricia averaged about five to six pounds a week. Determination and commitment to do everything possible to control her weight were what helped her. She is still averaging about three pounds a week. Her menstrual cycles are regular and not heavy, and there are no signs of precancerous uterine cells. She recently told me she feels like a new person, and although it was hard work, it was not as hard as she imagined it would be. She really believed that she was somehow different and unable to lose weight. Changing her attitude has spilled into different areas of her life as well. Where she previously felt certain things were unattainable, she now is figuring out how to achieve them.

The Basics of BMI

Body mass index, or BMI, is a number calculated from your weight and height. Although it has limitations, BMI is used by doctors and nutritionists as a way to estimate your general health. You can roughly calculate your BMI by using the chart in the Additional Resources section, or get the exact number at www.popweightloss. com.

Once you have your number, refer to this table to see if you fall within the healthy range.

Weight	Status
Below 18.5	Underweight
18.5 – 24.9	Normal
25.0 – 29.9	Overweight
30.0 – 34.9	Obese
35.0 and Above	Morbidly Obese

CHAPTER 7

JOSEPH, GRADUAL WEIGHT GAIN

Age: 46
Height: 5'11"
Weight Pre-Pop: 220 pounds
Current Weight: 175 pounds
Occupation: Physician and CEO of Healthy Woman OB/GYN and Pop Weight Loss
Relationship Status: Married for 16 years to a gorgeous OB/GYN and weight management physician (who might just be the author of this book!); one fantastic daughter, age 7

My husband, Joseph, is a very typical type A personality: an overachiever and entrepreneur who despite running two large and successful companies is always looking for his next challenge. He is intense and expects a lot from our co-workers, me, and our daughter. He is not the kind of person you can tell what to do; he must figure things out for himself.

Having said that, around the birth and first few years of our daughter's life, Joe's waistline was expanding. As an obstetrician, this is not unusual for me to see. Too many of my patients' husbands are overweight. During my pregnancy, my husband was in the kitchen with me routinely eating spaghetti and meatballs and large bowls of ice cream. My 50 pounds with pregnancy turned into 45 pounds for him. When I started the weight loss program and began to get healthy, he was supportive emotionally, but it took a while longer for his awakening moment to come. That happened when my daughter's fourth birthday party pictures came back — people are very funny about pictures and their weight, and I've found that pictures can be highly motivating. I put the photos in an album and was liking the way I looked, because even though I wasn't completely to my goal weight, the post-pregnancy blob me was gone. Joe, on the other hand, *hated* the pictures. He stared at them and said, "Do I really look like that? I have turned into my father." Joe's dad struggles badly with weight issues. He had quadruple bypass at age 59 and in his early 70s has a laundry list of medications and medical conditions. Joe was finally concerned about and aware of his weight being a health threat, and as a person who takes pride in his appearance, he was unhappy with the way he looked.

Right around this same time, my husband's blood pressure started going up, and we both knew where he was headed if he did not make some changes.

PRESCRIPTION

Once again, Joe's weight problems were a combination of the big Pop three: food, schedule, and a lack of exercise. Joe's schedule of eating was probably his No. 1 offender. At the time, he was a big meal skipper. I always say that if you skip a meal, you will make it up later and worse.

Joe would regularly drink coffee all day and most days have no real solid food until dinner at about 6 o'clock. Then because he had skipped breakfast and lunch, he was hungry all night and would snack the rest of the evening. When you eat late at night, you do not give your digestive system a chance to rest, you don't sleep well, and you are not hungry in the morning. It's a vicious cycle. Getting Joe to have breakfast with me and our daughter, Colette, at 6:30 a.m. was a major feat. He did not like my high-protein cereal or oatmeal but did settle on plain Cheerios, almonds, and berries. Dark berries like blueberries and blackberries are chocked with antioxidants and linked with benefits to men's health in particular.

Other food-related challenges with Joe included getting him away from sandwiches, pastries, and a lot of meat. The carbohydrates in white breads, sandwich rolls, and pastries raise our blood sugar too quickly, leading to weight gain and eventually diabetes. When I look back now, Joe ate too many breads and pastries. He still enjoys his pastries in moderation, and only if he feels they are truly worth eating.

With heart disease in his family, Joe had to get more fish into his diet. This was hard for him because meat really was a mainstay of his diet and he truly loves good food. He was never excited to order fish in a restaurant but now knows the importance. Omega-3 fatty acids reduce cholesterol and lower blood pressure — both of which are good for the heart — and are also helpful for skin and even mood. The highest omega-3 fatty acids come from salmon, sardines, anchovies, and walnuts. We had to keep trying different ways to incorporate more omega-3s and vegetarian items into Joe's diet. He now eats smoked salmon regularly, Cento Tuna from Italy (packed in olive oil, which is okay if you are using it as part of your dressing), lentil soup, and most fish. Another big factor concerning Joe's eating habits is that he is an excellent chef. Knowing that he could make the food taste better with more butter or bacon was a struggle for him, but the rewards of losing weight proved worth it.

Joe has also miraculously become an amazing runner who runs about five to six miles before work most days. Although he was a runner in high school, he was not very athletic in his adult life until this point. I am always asking people to find their inner athletic interest even if they never ran or played tennis before. Joe has a whole Zen-like routine that involves 300 push-ups and 500 sit-ups. He's made this exercise time his "me" time, and the difference in his stress level is amazing. Lucky for me, my husband's body is beyond a doubt better now than when we were married 16 years ago. I really do believe that not only is weight loss the true medicine, but it is the link to a great sex life. (No more to come on that subject!)

OUTCOME

Joe has lost 45 pounds, and his waist went from a size 38 to a size 32. He tells me it's all the little changes that add up to make weight loss a lifestyle change. He also says that he's addicted to the compliments from patients, friends, and co-workers he has not seen in a while. This can be very inspiring. Joe and I spend considerable time monitoring the health of our patients. We really do practice what we preach, and I believe it makes a big difference. I have friends who are weight loss doctors who are very overweight and unhealthy. I cannot see how they are believable to their patients. Most mornings Joe holds his hands up over his head as we get dressed and asks, "Am I not beautiful?" and I say, "Yes, you are beautiful." And he is.

6 Ways to Stay Heart-Healthy

Keeping your heart in excellent condition is important for everyone, but you should work all the harder at it if you have a history of heart disease in your family, as Joe does. Here are six things you can do:

- Reduce the saturated fats, cholesterol, and salt in your diet
- Get to — and stay at — a healthy weight
- Include fiber in your diet from fresh fruits and vegetables, beans, and seeds
- Monitor your blood pressure and blood cholesterol
- Limit the amount of alcohol you drink
- Get at least 30 minutes of cardiovascular exercise a day

EAT PLAN **MIND** BODY

There's no denying that weight loss is a process that involves many facets of your life. I've mentioned before that the foundation of Pop Weight Loss lies in three basic principles: food, schedule, and exercise. But behind all three of these is another important component: the psychological one.

My father recently told me that he went to a meeting where 1,000 people were assembled, most of them 50 to 80 years old, and about 85 percent were overweight or obese, according to his eyeball estimate. You probably have similar stories, and statistics back up the anecdotal evidence that obesity is indeed an epidemic today.

I bring up my father because he's a clinical psychologist who maintained an active practice for more than five decades, and he is constantly helping others, from the thousands of patients he's counseled over the years to a drowning nun he pulled from the water on the first day of his honeymoon. He's a strong positive force in the lives of our family and everyone who meets him. I'm constantly reminded of his easy-to-remember advice, and his words "think positive thoughts" ring in my ears daily. He believes it's his destiny to assist people, and I can't disagree with that. Fortunately, that desire to help extends to those who want to lose weight, and his insights on the psychological aspects of reaching your weight loss goals are invaluable.

In this section, my father, Dr. Kenneth Herman, will, in his own words, give you the psychological tools you need to overcome the many hurdles on the way to weight loss. With his insight into what makes people behave the way they do combined with the information in this book on eating right and exercising, you will have a complete toolkit for getting to the weight you want to be.

* * *

I was the worst student from kindergarten through high school. It was not until I was drafted into the Army in World War II that I discovered I was smarter than led to believe by my guidance counselor, who repeatedly told me to quit school and go to work. "School is not for you" was the guidance I received. I excelled as a student in college and graduated undergraduate school in three years. My master's degree at Boston University and a doctorate at Columbia University followed. I have also studied at Harvard, The New School, New York University, and the State University of Iowa. In 2001 after 9/11 at the age of 74, I took courses in aviation crises management training and post-trauma intervention training. In 2004, I completed another trauma training course. I am always amazed with how much I still have to learn.

I consider myself fortunate to have discovered my passion for helping people. My destiny has been to make the world better and I have had unlimited opportunities to see that become a reality. I maintained an active practice for 50 years. Upon retiring, I published a personal growth book called *Secrets from the Sofa* that has helped many. I serve on the board of trustees of a free medical center that treats the uninsured. I am part of a group that is making medical miracles happen each day.

I am often asked what motivated me to be a psychologist. In my first year of college, I declared my major to be psychology. Certainly at that time at 20 years of age I did not know about the arduous academic road ahead to attain that goal. What I did know is the personal satisfaction of helping another person to cope more effectively and feel better. I seek out situations where my human relations skills can be of help — and aiding people to get in the right mind-set for losing weight is one of those.

For example, while attending a party some time ago, I sat down with a lady I know. The woman is overweight and was eating a creamy cake delight. She asked if I wanted one. When I declined and told her it would be too difficult to work off, she replied: "I don't have the willpower not to eat it." Glad to have the opportunity to talk to her about losing weight, I told her about protecting her health. I also mentioned that she's very attractive and would look spectacular if she made an effort to lose weight. A few months later, I saw her again at another party. The first thing she said to me was: "Since we last talked, I've lost nine pounds. Sometimes a little encouragement goes a long way."

Those are the kind of interactions that inspire me, and I hope that by sharing what I've learned during my career and lifetime, I can help you realize the same success.

CHAPTER 8

DECIDING TO CHANGE

Perhaps the most important thing to know from a mental standpoint about losing weight is this: It is always possible to change. You may have factors working against you — a busy schedule, obesity in the family, a love of sweets, an injury — but it's always possible to turn it around. You have to truly believe that. As you've read in the case studies that opened this book, people from all walks of life and with all kinds of different issues have found a way to change — and you can, too. Many of my patients feel that they are somehow different, and despite being successful in other aspects of their lives, they feel that they cannot get control of their weight. This is simply not true.

If your body, health, and appearance are important to you, Dr. Rebecca and I are here to help. We will point you in the direction toward a slender body, greater pep and energy, better sex, and an improved way of life. The end product of all this will elevate your feelings about yourself. We can't do it without your help. You are the star in the show. We need you to look forward to the lifetime rewards of being healthy. I have seen so many people in my office and my gym get into physically better shape and then go on to other achievements. One man got in such good shape that he landed a position he formerly only could dream about. Success in many settings requires that people make a good appearance. This is the time for you to take charge of your life.

In preparation for writing this section, I checked some of the weight reduction books on the market. Many of them provide exercises for readers to do concerning their eating habits. We are not requesting you answer too many questions because we know from vast experience what our readers are thinking and what they are seeking from reading a book like this. Therefore, we are cutting to the chase to make it crystal clear for you to lose weight and adapt permanent good eating habits without much delay. We are recommending you change your thinking habits about eating and go in the direction of being optimistic. We require you to get rid of any assumptions about yourself as a person that are not positive. Remember, if others can control their weight, you can, too. It is imperative that you recognize your strengths. If anything in your life is holding you back from feeling stable and emotionally secure, let's deal with it so you are in a good frame of mind to face life's challenges directly. We want you to have peace of mind. We want you to anticipate that you will finally feel you have a plan you can follow. You are in the driver's seat. You can make it happen. Check your confidence meter. We need it to be on the right side of your confidence meter gauge. Don't anticipate failure just because it has happened repeatedly before.

Every person reading this matters a great deal. And while you are special in many ways, remember that you are no different than anyone else trying to tackle the problem of weight loss. You *can* reach your goals. In the next section, Dr. Rebecca will give you very specific steps to get to where you want to be, but first, you have to be in the right frame of mind.

If you are reading this book, you may be more motivated than you think. Your curiosity brought you to explore why you are overweight. Maybe your clothes are too tight. Maybe a look in the mirror terrified you. Maybe someone commented that you've gained weight. Maybe you know someone who lost weight with this program and had success. Many people just reach a point where the weight is too painful to ignore any longer. Whatever it is, you know it is time for concern. Whether you visited your doctor or came to this book on your own, you are searching for solutions and that is a good sign. Whatever your reasons, welcome aboard.

IMAGINING A NEW LIFE

If you could magically push a button and select to weigh a certain weight, think of what that weight would be. Now that you have that particular number in mind, picture how you would look. Do you like what you see in your mind's eye? Now think of the benefits that you would derive from that ideal weight. Would you go out socially with more enthusiasm because of the way you look or dress? Do you feel any better about yourself? Do you think you have protected your health status? Are you proud of your accomplishment? Do you think your friends and family see you in a different light?

Continue to picture yourself at the ideal weight you magically established. Has your lifestyle changed? Are you feeling any more energetic as you go through your day? Do you have any more drive to do housework or chores requiring physical strength? Do you find yourself getting more accomplished? Are you less tired during the day?

Imagine that along with your ideal weight, you are exercising daily. Imagine looking forward to this time as your special time. Imagine seeing exercise in a whole different light and accomplishing things physically that you haven't done in years or were never able to do. Picture your pride in putting in the effort to arrive at your ideal weight. Visualize yourself in good shape feeling stronger and less fatigued. Picture yourself adopting the healthy food and exercise habits forever and living life to its fullest.

If you are reaping all these benefits, why wouldn't you continue to eat healthy and exercise? Now remember the tired feelings and medical problems that come with an unhealthy weight. Imagine never going back to your old habits of losing weight and gaining it back. How are you feeling about having controlled your weight and being physically in shape, even if it was in your mind's eye? Pretty good, I am guessing.

The reason for asking you to imagine what life could be like for you is that it is possible for you to go from imagining to really making permanent changes with your eating and exercise habits. It is true that many people fail to stay with a sound eating and exercise plan. But Dr. Rebecca and I are asking you to be an eagle and not fly with the flock. We are asking you to use all your strength to finally take charge of your life and follow our lead.

In the course of each day, you think and do many things. If you don't believe me, write down your thoughts and actions for a given day. You will be amazed. Lots of thinking and behavior takes place. We are asking you to make sure your thinking and actions coincide with your commitment to eat healthy and exercise. We want this trip toward health to be different from all other failed attempts. We want this book to be your chance to truly make a difference in your life. We want you to believe in yourself and know that you have the ability to be successful. If you can solidify the image of the person you want to be and imagine this person first thing in the morning and at night as you're going to sleep, this person will become a reality.

THE ESSENTIALS TO THINK ABOUT

Losing weight is a combination of changing physically and mentally. Here's what you need to keep in mind:

1. Understand there is a need to change your eating habits
2. Identify the unhealthy foods to avoid
3. Bring healthier foods into your life
4. Realize good feelings and better health stem from a true commitment to change
5. Realize that exercising will help the stresses in your life and keep your weight off long term

Dismiss the idea of being on or off a diet. One meal, one day, one week, one month does not matter. Staying on the path to health long term is the only thing that matters.

The other sections of this book give you an eating template and show you the kind of foods you need to fuel your body, but how do you solidify that now is the time to change and that doing so can only bring benefits? Becoming healthier can improve your life in so many ways you may not yet realize.

Take, for example, Irma, a 40-year-old executive assistant to a corporate attorney who was referred to me because of anxiety attacks. As she came to terms with her fears and became more confident, she lost 49 pounds. Here's what she said afterward:

"You taught me that the anxiety causing my problems was really because I was afraid of so many things. When you told me to assert myself, I thought you were making me worse. You made me confront my boss and I thought I was going to lose my job. I couldn't believe he gave me a raise and started to treat me nicer. You told me to use the anxiety as a signal that something in my life needs to be faced. When I get anxious now, I can pretty much tell what is bothering me and figure out what to do. That makes me feel stronger. To be honest, I never thought I would lose weight. I had tried so many times before and nothing happened. I guess I was eating without thinking about it, putting on extra pounds. I am more careful about what I eat and take more pride in how I look."

Or listen to the story of May, a 37-year-old secretary of a fellow psychologist. Her boss asked me if I would speak with her because she continued to get into unrewarding relationships. A few weeks after she stopped coming in for therapy, she sent me this letter:

"I wasn't proud of being overweight but never thought it was the reason I was not particular with whom I dated. I used to think I was lucky to get someone to take me out. No wonder I wasn't selective. It all sounds so simple now that I am stronger. It is funny — my job brings me in touch with anxious, depressed people, but I never thought too much about what sort of person I was. When you asked me to make a list of my strengths, I was speechless. 'What strengths?' I thought. When you told me everybody has strengths, it started me thinking. Holy smokes! To think what I have learned after living all these years is amazing. And to have lost weight, too, is really a bonus. I haven't found the man I am looking for yet, but at least I know he is out there."

Or consider Mike, a 39-year-old bank manager who came to see me because he was compulsively eating. He was planning to marry and felt he owed it to himself and his fiancée to trim down. Not only did he improve his relationship, he also started excelling in other areas. After six months of therapy and 53 pounds lost, he said:

"My boss paid me a compliment the other day. He said I am more organized and professional. He likes the way I represent the bank. The big thing I want to say to you is that Michelle is so proud of the changes I have made. Don't get me wrong, Doc — she liked me before as a potential husband, but now I can see she is really proud to be with me. Of course that makes me happy."

None of these people came to me confident that they could lose weight, and none came specifically for weight loss. As they progressed along their journey, though, they began to believe they could do it — and that is a crucial step.

We have not complicated the content of this book with many statistics or studies substantiating the harmful effects of neglecting your health if you fail to eat healthy and exercise. You probably know all the danger signs. Real medical problems come to people who ignore their weight. It is foolish to assume you are immune to the life-threatening health problems that stem from poor eating habits and lack of exercise. What can happen to someone else can happen to you and me.

Carl was referred to me because of having high blood pressure. Here is what he had to say: "I am here because my doctor thinks I am too nervous. To tell you the truth, I admit to being the nervous type but seem to get by all right. Whenever I feel the pressure of business or whatever is bothering me, I go out and buy a few suits or go on a cruise and I feel better. It is my way of dealing with stress. To be honest with you, I don't believe in taking problems to a therapist. Anybody who can't handle his own issues is weak. Life is tough and if you can't handle the day-to-day problems, you're going to sink." Carl had his own solutions to resolving the stresses in his life: You just push them under the rug, buy new clothes, and go on a cruise. Unfortunately, Carl had a massive heart attack and died at the age of 57. That is a sad but true story. The consequences of neglecting your health can be fatal — you cannot afford to ignore it.

This is a tough lesson that I'm still heartbroken to say one of my childhood friends never grasped. He smoked all his life and would tell me how many gifts he received from Raleigh cigarette coupons. He also was at least 100 pounds overweight throughout his adult life. I talked to him numerous times about quitting smoking and losing weight. He would say telling him to stop smoking and lose weight was like him telling me not to work so many hours. He retired with a nice pension from a big corporation and talked about getting into a fun and profitable venture with me. While he was typing a letter to me, he had a fatal heart attack. His wife forwarded me the letter. It said: "I appreciate your keeping after me to stop smoking and lose weight. I am not proud of my overeating and smoking. I know both the habits are harmful. I deserve your criticism and harmful effects from both habits." He thought he deserved the harmful effects but never thought the combination of smoking and obesity would kill him. My friend was only 60 years old. He was smart and had many talents but didn't use his good mind to prolong his life.

You don't have to follow the same path that so many other people do. The fact that you're reading this puts you ahead of the game, and we're going to equip you with the tools you need to reach your goals.

CHAPTER 9

HOW TO KNOW YOU CAN SUCCEED THIS TIME

If you're like most people, you've probably tried and failed in the past to maintain a healthy lifestyle over the long term. If it were easy, no one would struggle with weight problems. But it's also not as difficult as you may think. It does, however, take one crucial element: You have to want it. Do you?

It is wonderful that you are reading this book, but it would really be terrific knowing that you are highly motivated and will act to complete this transformation. Take this quiz below to ascertain your motivation to be successful this time. On a five-point scale, where do you rate? One is slightly motivated and five is highly motivated.

	1	2	3	4	5
I want to lose weight					
I will put effort into changing					
I will be patient to reach my goal					
I will be successful this time					
I will not eat poorly when stressed					
I will make exercise a priority					
I will be careful not to overeat					
I will stay away from junk food					

Does this quiz give you an idea of how motivated you are to lose weight? If you told yourself you're ready to make the necessary changes, I am happy for you. It is said that the truth about how good the pudding is is in the tasting. If you truly feel this is your time to change, *make it happen*! I'll be there at the finish line to cheer you on.

THIS TIME *CAN* BE DIFFERENT

Most people who pick up a book like this automatically think that what they are going to read is old hat. You might be thinking you have tried all these ideas before. You might be thinking you don't really eat that much food. You may be pessimistic about anything changing for you. I give you full credit for all you have done in the past to change. However, if you still have not achieved your goals, you cannot continue to do what is making you unhappy. Whatever you've tried in the past has not been enough. My daughter Dr. Rebecca tells us eating healthy foods in the right proportions, regular exercise, and a set schedule will make you lose weight and improve your health. I will tell you that being confident and having good coping mechanisms to deal with life's stresses are just as important. You need to change your thinking to be receptive to a new plan. What has transpired in the past need not interfere with your success this time.

I am not concerned if you failed to control your weight previously. It only means you have not committed to a healthy plan before, or maybe it wasn't the right time for you. This is a different time and an opportunity to learn a new way to approach and resolve your weight concerns. Follow my lead and you will discover new skills. You need to believe in your ability. Eating foods that are in your best interest can be great to restore your energy and really quite enjoyable. Your newfound way of eating will not take anything away but only add pleasure to your life. In fact, knowing you are protecting your health will give you a new sense of security.

If you have a history of not being able to control your weight, it is easy to see why you may be pessimistic regarding your ability to change. You are conditioned to fail. A major league baseball player made an appointment to see me because he was in a batting slump. I was surprised to see him and wondered how many people in the waiting room recognized him. He told me he was getting up to the plate with a negative attitude. "I have struck out so many times, I expect to strike out," he commented.

I told him what Tom Seaver said about not dwelling on the numbers. He said that was all well and good, but if he continued to strike out, he would be gone. Under hypnosis I suggested that he forget the fact that he was recently hitting poorly and recall that he was a recognized major league player with an excellent record. I reminded him that he was knowledgeable about the game and aware of what he had to do to start hitting again. I told him that the next time he was at bat, he would have a more positive attitude and be confident about getting a hit. The very next game he got a single and a double. Hypnosis is not magic. I was able to appeal to him to approach the plate with a more confident mind-set.

This Hall of Fame baseball player shows us that what you think does influence your being successful or failing. I know that many people have tried numerous diet programs and failed. If every time you picked up a particular pencil, the lead broke, you would get to the point where you would chuck the pencil whenever you picked it up. Your past failed attempts may be discouraging or at least make you question if you can successfully control your weight and life. Remember, if it is humanly possible and others do it, so can you. You are no different. If you can make up your mind to be successful and see yourself as the person you want to be, you will be successful.

Intellectually, you want to lose weight, but it has not happened. You feel lousy about your inability to succeed. You think of yourself as a failure — like the baseball player. If you have not been able to lose weight, try not to put yourself down in any way. It is not in your best interest to think poorly of yourself. Forgive yourself. You should not beat yourself up about past failures. You must move forward. Maybe you have not found the approach that will work for you until now.

The good news is the ballgame is not over. You are not a failure. We are with you to urge you to continue trying. We will fortify you with the encouragement and a plan for eating well. Don't make your task any more complicated than it is. Many individuals over-complicate the process or give up too quickly. Know in your mind that you are not wimpy and this time you are going to be able to achieve your goals. The rewards of wellness are far greater than the feelings of failure. Change is scary and resistance to change is normal. You might say you want to change, but if your behavior doesn't match your words, then you are only staying with what is safe and comfortable. You may think you don't have the discipline to change, but you do. Have faith in your ability to make the commitment to change. When you do, it will elevate your self-esteem. It is when you are feeling the power of self-confidence that you will experience real strength to make decisions you didn't think you could.

When treating young people, I would often play chess during the therapy session. Playing chess provides many opportunities to teach children what to do when faced with conflict. For example, I would tell the child there are three things to do when a chess piece is threatened. One could take the opponent's piece if possible, one could hide for protection behind his or her piece, or one could escape. Then I would ask the patient if there were any choices regarding what to do about resolving the conflict he or she was experiencing. Often the child would mention a resolution not thought of before. Remember, past failures aren't important because there is always a second chance at being successful.

Learn from your mistakes and move forward. We all have the potential to be successful if we persevere. Resistance to success is to be expected but need not be a barrier to change. Each barrier you face on your journey to health is an opportunity to learn from your mistakes and come back stronger.

TAKE A GOOD LOOK AT WHAT'S GOING ON IN YOUR LIFE

Some questions I raised when writing my last book, *Secrets from the Sofa*, centered around people reaching for happiness. If what everyone really wants from life is happiness, success, and peace of mind, then why do people stay at unrewarding jobs or in destructive relationships? Why are people neglecting their physical and mental health? Why do we sometimes have trouble getting through the day? Unfortunately, people feel safe and secure with familiar emotions. Even misery can be preferable to the anticipated anxiety associated with change. Intellectually, we would like to change; emotionally, we question if change is necessary or even possible.

A good place to start is by writing a log and taking a personal inventory. I've often requested my patients do this because it's a good way for people to think about who they are and what changes they would like to make in their life. Try writing about your childhood and what you remember. How would you describe your relationship with your parents and siblings? Who were the important people in your life? What were your school experiences? Write about your interests and thoughts about life. Write about your dreams and aspirations. What do you consider your strong and weak points? How would you like to change? What do you think of your eating habits? What are your goals concerning food? How motivated are you to lose weight forever? How would you describe yourself emotionally? How do you think other people see you? Are you troubled about any particular problems? Name three wishes. Do you have any regrets? Do you feel guilty about anything? Whom would you really like to be? List your attributes. If you take this task seriously, you will recall a lot of information that will have meaning for you.

You may realize you have some issues in your life you need to deal with. Throughout the years, I kept notes about my patients and reviewed them for research projects and lessons learned. I always made note if my patients were struggling with their weight. What became obvious to me is that those patients who lost weight and did not regain those extra pounds were the ones who made significant progress in other areas of their life. Maybe they resolved conflict with a boss or friend, maybe they finally got out of a bad relationship, or maybe they got the courage to leave a job that was unrewarding. There is a strong connection between improving your life in general and gaining control of your life — including your exercise and eating habits.

Knowing that you will be successful losing weight if you check for unresolved issues in your life and face them should give you a new approach to getting healthy. As a psychologist, I am encouraging you to focus on all aspects of your life because your chances of success losing weight will be greater. You might feel that you're not signing up for therapy; you only want to lose weight. There is a natural resistance to change, and we know people are prone to stay with what is safe and comfortable. It's tough to face what you might fear. However, whenever you have the guts to face what you fear, that fear will be reduced. You may be anxious facing the truth or addressing a problem, but when you do, that fear will be abated. Additionally, you will be proud of yourself for being assertive.

If you are troubled with anxiety, depression, guilt, phobias, or anger, remember that turning to food will not make you feel better in the long run. People often comfort themselves with food because of unresolved emotional issues. I want you to learn other activities that bring comfort or joy to your life. I believe that these unresolved issues account for the percentage of people benefiting from weight reduction programs being so low. Even when weight is lost, 80 percent of people regain weight after a year. These statistics are not seen on this program. We believe the reason is that this program is a true lifestyle change. Just as important as your eating healthy foods and exercising is your examining the messages you send to yourself, what is unresolved in your life, and other issues that may be making you unhappy. The stronger you become emotionally, the greater the probability of success with reaching all your health goals.

I want you to hear Carolyn's story because she once had many doubts about her ability to lose weight. I saw her as a person with a lot of potential for change and therefore encouraged her to continue to see me. Carolyn is 42, married with two children. Prior to marriage, she worked as a nurse at a hospital in New

York City. She had a successful career but stopped working to take care of her children. When not attending to family chores, she was active in church and community affairs.

Carolyn grew up in the Midwest in a small Iowa city on a farm. After college, she married and moved to Boston. She said her childhood was good and that she was a happy person. She never had a problem with weight until she got married, when she gradually gained a significant amount of weight. She was upset with herself that she was overweight because she certainly knew her weight could lead to all kinds of health problems. However, she did not seem to be able to stay with a plan for losing weight. A lot of times, knowing you need to lose weight is not enough — success is not in the knowing but the doing. She thought seeing a psychologist might give her the motivation she was seeking.

Sometimes a psychologist has to listen with a third ear to understand the meaning that might be behind what a patient is saying. Carolyn did not acknowledge any specific problem areas in her life. However, we both thought her inability to take the weight off must be indicative of some frustration in her life. Carolyn said, "My marriage is good and I love being a mother. I always wanted to be part of a family and thought that this lifestyle would make me happy. I must admit I loved being a nurse and thought of going to medical school; I was pre-med in college. When I graduated college, nursing school seemed like a natural road for me because I was dating Dan at the time and we planned on getting married. My biology professor at Cornell was disappointed I didn't apply to medical school."

I asked Carolyn how she felt not pursuing medical school. She continued, "I can't say I didn't think of it. In fact, it comes up in my dreams. Once in a while, when I was in the operating room, I would think that I could do what the doctors were doing. With the proper training, I could really see myself being a doctor."

Carolyn admitted she was thinking about working soon because the children did not need her as much. Although she most likely would return to nursing, she asked if I thought she was too old to try to get into medical school. I continued to see Carolyn once a week for several months. We did not talk specifically about her weight, but she told me she had joined an exercise group at the Y and was paying more attention to what she was eating. She thought she had lost a few pounds.

Carolyn continued to be enthusiastic about coming to see me. She was eager to talk about her plans to return to work. She came to the conclusion that she would not pursue medical school but be happy if she could be back in the operating room. The hospital where she had worked was eager for her to return.

I cannot specifically tell you what enabled Carolyn to feel more relaxed, lose weight, join an exercise program, and generally be more pleased with herself, but it gradually was happening. Coming to see me and taking stock of what was going on in her life enabled her to sort matters out and get on a healthy road. Possibly she was not completely satisfied at home and began to eat as a means of seeking pleasure from food. Her weight was a sign to her that all was not well.

I wasn't surprised to see that Carolyn was happier and making good plans for the future because I have seen this type of progress many times. People are often considerably more capable of dealing with life's obstacles than they give themselves credit for. In Carolyn's case, she responded favorably to the intervention of therapy, but therapy is not always necessary. This book has an ample amount of ammunition to help individuals eat wisely and exercise. It will require an assessment of your life to ascertain how you can think and act on your best behalf. It will require that you identify any unresolved problems so you are not at risk of emotional eating. It will require you to find solutions to the normal problems of life. You will need to sort through your emotions and explore if you are eating because you are actually hungry, or if it's because you're sad, depressed, anxious, frustrated, or bored. This idea can be very liberating. It will require you are in the good frame of mind to make the best effort at eating on a schedule, exercising, and choosing healthy foods. This is your chance to shine and be successful.

PINPOINTING YOUR MOTIVATION

Whenever a new patient came to see me, I always listened carefully to understand the problems being presented and simultaneously make an assessment of the person's receptivity to change. Some people deny the existence of problems and others are so defensive that their mind is closed to change. If the patient is seeking help because of being overweight, I might ask how the weight problem currently affects his or her life. I recently spoke to an overweight man who told me he has no problem living with his weight. He is not likely to be interested in eating properly or exercising. If I hear that the person is concerned because of feeling embarrassed about his or her weight, fearful of illness, or soon needing an operation if weight is not lost, I know that the person will be motivated to change and that losing weight is considered important.

I then inquire about what people have done to date to resolve the problem. Have they seen other professionals? I want to know if they have entered into weight-reducing programs before and how successful they were. If the program did not meet their expectations, I want to know what happened. I want to see what we can learn from previous attempts. Carlo told me he has gained weight because his wife serves a lot of food and he doesn't want to refuse to eat for fear of hurting her feelings. He knows that his thinking is faulty and that his weight problem will remain the same or get worse. If you are making excuses, listen to and learn from the messages you are sending to yourself.

You will see throughout this section that there is a lot of information to motivate and stimulate you to be successful this time. Keep in mind if others have done it, you can, too. To help you start to make permanent changes, I want you to make a list of what it would mean to you to lose weight. Here is what being in shape means to me:

1. Eating foods that are nutritious affords me good health in my mid-80s
2. I like the proud messages I send to myself when I see I look good
3. I like the fact that clothes fit and look great on me
4. As a professional person, my appearance enhances the respect people have for me and enables me to be more effective in motivating my patients
5. I equate being healthy with being alive — really living life to the fullest and not having to turn down invitations because I'm tired or sick
6. I have more energy being in good physical condition
7. I know if I get sick, being healthy will result in a faster recovery
8. I am more mentally alert
9. My family and friends are pleased to see me taking care of myself

Now how about your list? Don't you want to be that person at the wedding or high school reunion who looks fantastic? I hope that making your list will allow you to realize the long-term benefits of getting healthy. Living a healthy life results in a multitude of rewards for each of us. Give some thought to your list and refer to it every week. It will keep you motivated to succeed. Place it next to a picture of yourself that you really like or a picture of what you would really like to look like.

Staying motivated also requires sending yourself positive messages — negativity is not helpful when it comes to pushing yourself to make a life change. Send positive messages to yourself and avoid self-criticism. Focus on your strengths and create a meaningful life by developing many interests. Each time you do something new, you add a new dimension to your personality. It is most important that you set realistic goals. Trying to replace negative habits with those that are healthy takes time. Be pleased you are making progress and going in the right direction.

Also try to diminish any negative influences in your life. If a friend or support person is not happy for you that you are making changes in your life for the better, you may need to re-evaluate that relationship. Any truly loving and positive person in your life would only want you to be the best person you can be. If you feel you have no time at all to spend on yourself, it is time to take a hard look at all of your commitments to see which ones can be eliminated or reduced. Just like negative relationships, work or family commitments that negatively influence you or your time should be minimized.

I coached little league baseball for many years. Most of the youngsters were grade-school age, and when I wanted to make the important point not to leave the base early, I would ask them to send the message to their brain that they cannot leave the base until the ball is pitched. It is the brain that is the chief commander of all we think and do. I have the same message for people who are concerned about getting healthy. Let it register in your mind that you will do all possible to pay special attention to what you eat, your schedule, and your exercise habits. Reading this book is the path to developing a new way of thinking about your body. Your brain will be your protector to make sure you are applying all the new information you are learning about healthy eating. Here are the messages regarding your weight that will be best for you to send to your brain:

1. will think about what I am going to eat prior to eating
2. I will select healthy foods such as fruits and vegetables, nuts and beans, and fish and chicken
3. I will be conscious of not overeating
4. I will avoid junk food and prepackaged food as much as possible
5. I will make an effort to stick to my eating schedule
6. I will control my eating one day at a time and develop a new relationship with food
7. I will deal with my personal problems and not eat under stress
8. I will be conscious of food traps
9. I will take pride in controlling my weight
10. I will be patient to reach my weight goals
11. I will not go back to my poor eating habits even if my progress is slow
12. I will treat myself the best way I can
13. I will take advantage of this opportunity forever
14. I will practice only good eating habits
15. I will make exercise a habit
16. I will recognize my strengths often and avoid self-criticism
17. I will aspire to be the person of my dreams
18. I will think of food for health instead of food for comfort
19. I will surround myself with positive people who are also living a healthy lifestyle
20. I will balance out each day
21. If I stray from eating healthily, I will immediately regroup

YOU'RE WORTH IT

One of the most difficult obstacles to helping people is to sell confidence and self-respect to a person who does not feel worthy. Individuals who have been rejected or abused often do not feel they are entitled to success. They are usually self-critical and at times self-destructive. If you are not emotionally secure and have feelings of inadequacy, it will be essential for you to feel better about yourself so that you can treat yourself well. I will go so far as to say your gaining feelings of self-worth is a prerequisite to your losing weight permanently. Unless you respect yourself and treat yourself well, you will be unlikely to feel worthy of getting healthy. You must see yourself as a person worthy of change.

I never told a patient struggling with life's many issues that resolving problems is easy. Whether we are talking about losing weight, dealing with a sexual problem, coping with marital conflict, or handling guilt, life can be most complicated. One of my friends, Dr. Daniel Sugarman, an eminent psychologist and author of *The Search for Serenity*, stresses that individuals who are confident and have good coping skills seem to control their life. The best weight reduction program in the world will take perseverance and self-confidence to realize success. If you believe in yourself, you will succeed.

YOUR VIRTUAL VISIT

Consider reading this book like an opportunity to sit down with Dr. Rebecca and me. Here is what we probably would discuss. We know you are concerned about your weight (unless you are reading this book to seek help for a loved one). We would be telling you that this is your opportunity to get healthy. Most of the patients who have come to us for help with weight loss are skeptical that it will work for them. We know, too, from a great deal of experience that you are probably not optimistic about losing weight even now. Few people who are concerned about weight think they can change. We expect doubt and we expect resistance to change. If you have reservations about being able to lose weight, *you are normal!* The reason you are normal is that most people who try to lose weight fail and give up too easily. They are pessimistic about achieving their goals and use the slightest setback to give up. I have heard my daughter tell patients and family members one day or one week or even one month of being off track with diet or exercise does not matter. It is the concept of being on a journey and staying with it for the long haul to get healthy that is important.

We are optimistic you can change. I'll tell you why we're so optimistic. The content of this book is based on what has been effective with many people just like you. We hope that by sharing what transpired with our patients, you will be able to approach the task of getting healthier with less trepidation and greater confidence. Be assured that we're aware that many of you may be programmed to fail because you have not been as successful in the past. We know about how an overwhelming number of individuals lose weight and gain it back many times. We ask that you be patient to try again with a more positive attitude about changing. We can help if you are serious about changing.

Before starting any weight reduction program, we recommend you go to your primary care doctor for a checkup. Trying to get healthy for some people has been an elusive undertaking for which there appears to be no resolution. Patients have often told me of past failures despite their giving the matter their best effort. Although we are presenting information that should make a difference for readers, there are medical conditions that can slow metabolism.

Even if you have a medical condition that is slowing your progress, this is not a reason to give up. This time around it will work if you get serious about changing and being proud of yourself. Excess weight is something that we see whether we are standing in front of a mirror, lying in bed, or taking a shower. Our body is there to observe. Is it there to be proud of or ashamed of? You know the answer.

I give a lot of thought to why people have so much of a problem controlling their weight. Sure, there are plenty of food traps out there to entice folks to eat. But intelligent people know how to avoid them. We know that people primarily gain weight by eating too much food. If we take in more than we burn off, we are inviting extra pounds. There is nothing complicated about that. The Pop Weight Loss plan will give you excellent guidelines to follow, but that is not sufficient unless you change your behavior. Make this book the beginning of your lifestyle change. We will give you the information you need. We need you to change your behavior regarding how you process that information. Make this the time that you're ready to do that for good.

CHAPTER 10

MAKING A CHANGE

Now that you've decided you're ready to make a change and you know that this time, you can be successful, it's time to put in the work to get to your goals. While most people focus on the physical changes they make — adjusting their eating habits, workout routines, and sleep schedules — the psychological changes are just as important to keep in mind.

You must think positively about your journey to get healthy. Note the messages you are sending to yourself. Are they positive messages, or do you dread all the effort it will take? Positive messages are: "I equate eating healthy with avoiding a heart attack or getting diabetes" or "I am giving up desserts because they put on extra pounds I don't need." Negative messages are: "Life is too short to deny myself whatever gives me pleasure" or "I've tried many times to lose weight and you practically have to starve yourself." Keep your thoughts positive and it *will* make a difference.

EATING MINDFULLY

Once you're on board mentally with losing weight, one of the biggest struggles is changing your diet. That's why sticking to a plan is so helpful — if you're eating three meals and two snacks a day as Dr. Rebecca recommends, there's no time for emotional eating.

If you're anything like the average person, you engage in mindless eating that you may not be aware of. I just came from the supermarket and purchased grapes. While I was shopping, I must have eaten a dozen grapes. I committed a crime in more ways than one. We are so used to tasting what is in sight that we do unconscious eating time and time again. Enjoy food, but do it slowly, and only at snack time or mealtime. I want you to have more control over what and how much you eat. This book's main focus is on making you an informed person regarding your eating habits. There are forces in the world that are trying to influence you to eat all kinds of tasty foods. Corporations spend millions to attract consumers to their products. I want you to be an expert on controlling what you eat and censoring any messages designed to entice you.

I am sure we have all experienced eating leftover foods even though we weren't hungry. Maybe it was a few cold French fries. Maybe it was the crusty remains of an apple pie. Try to break yourself of feeling the need to eat whatever you see. If there is leftover food after you've eaten, put it in the refrigerator or throw it out. Send the message to your brain that it is not your job to be the cleanup person with foods remaining after the meal. Just as leftovers can be a danger zone, you may have other triggers for mindless eating. There was a time when I would go on a tasting spree sampling all my wife was making. "What the heck," I would think, "it's only a little bite." *It all adds up.*

When it comes to mealtime, be aware of how much food is on your plate. Usually we know how much it will take to make us satiated. Make a habit of taking a little less than filling up the entire plate, and eat until you are only 80 percent full, as the Japanese do. Many patients admit they are not hungry for meals because they are snacking throughout the day or eating while they are cooking. It will feel good to be hungry for a meal and be able to have the control to enjoy it slowly. Research shows that people who pre-plate their food eat less than people who go back again for more food. My daughter recommends eating one plate of food slowly. Remember her Dr. Rebecca 18-minute rule — your brain does not know you have eaten until 18 minutes have passed. So slow down, put your fork down between bites, and enjoy your meal. Consuming your portions quickly just leads to overeating.

Reading this book puts you in the position of eliminating surprises from your eating habits. We don't want you to be surprised that your dress or jeans are too tight or that you have a new medical problem. The way you will do it is by paying attention to all aspects of your life having to do with food — that means when you are shopping and wherever you are contemplating eating. Take the time to plan ahead and don't make the task complicated. If you care about your body, you will be careful to screen what goes into your mouth and ultimately make healthy choices automatically.

Be aware that whenever you are going out to dinner with friends or have an event like a wedding, you will probably be sitting and eating longer than when at home. A longer period at the dinner table lends itself to more eating unless you pace yourself. You don't have to eat all the food offered; be selective. Stick with the foods on the program. Offer to bring something if you're going to a friend's home for dinner and don't know what kind of food will be there.

Research also tells us that people who watch a lot of television are more likely to overeat than those who do not. A lot of unconscious eating takes place at all ages when people are concentrating on a TV program. Some folks would not think of watching television without all sorts of snacks on hand. A patient of mine, Tim, lost a good deal of weight when he and his wife removed all the junk food from the living room where they watch television.

He says: "It started with us bringing in a box of pretzels. Then it was crackers. Then we had the idea to get special containers for the different items. We both were putting on the weight and wondering where it was coming from. It creeps up on you. One day, my dad was over and couldn't believe all the food in the living room. At first we thought it would make watching TV more pleasant. We had all our favorite snacks. We have pretty good eating habits at mealtime. We were messing up big and didn't even realize it until gaining the extra weight. We got rid of it all. In fact, we now realize a lot of the things we had aren't even good to eat."

THE MIND-BODY CONNECTION

Another major component to weight loss is exercise. There's no way around it — if you want to change your life, it is necessary to add this component. We know emphatically that exercise is a key factor to losing weight and for long-term maintenance. If you haven't made exercise a priority, the weight will remain if you continue to pay little attention to an activity schedule. You must make a commitment to enter into an activity program, even if you need to start slowly. The daily habit is more important than the activity itself. If you are not motivated to exercise, you will undermine your efforts to lose weight no matter how much you change your eating habits. Albert Einstein once said: "Life is like riding a bicycle. To keep your balance, you must keep moving."

Years ago I decided to join a gym and exercise five days a week. I usually do my exercise early in the morning. If I have a meeting, I schedule the gym later. It is as important to me as bathing and brushing my teeth. That is the type of dedication to exercise that is needed to be healthy and to maintain weight loss. Attending a gym is not the only way to stay in shape. If a gym is not your choice, find some activity you enjoy. Run, walk, play tennis, swim, or participate in any other activity that helps you get a cardiovascular workout. Toning classes like Pilates and yoga, along with resistance activities such as weight training, are excellent choices once you get close to your goal weight, but it's the cardio habit that we need first.

I wouldn't do anything in my life that is not rewarding in some way — so I wouldn't expect you to, either. Find what it is about exercise that brings you the greatest benefits and pleasure. For me, it's staying healthy and mobile. I don't want to be plagued with a stroke, osteoporosis, diabetes, or cancer. Exercising keeps your heart in shape. I am certain my workout habit is keeping me from medical problems.

Another reason I exercise is that it's as important as eating correctly. The body demands it and responds negatively without it. A lack of exercise will result in becoming lethargic and old before your time. Exercising delays the aging process and keeps the muscles toned. People who exercise move about with greater mobility and ease and have a lower incidence of Alzheimer's disease, while people who shy away from physical activity take considerably more effort to go about their day. I watched a man take a stress test in the gym the other day. He was worn out before he started. He said he hadn't exercised for quite a while. I hope that he will now, as it's never too late to start — for him or you.

WHO SUCCEEDS — AND WHO DOESN'T?

People from all walks of life and all sets of circumstances can make this plan work for them. Those who are successful are selective in their choice of foods, are cognizant of the quantity of food they consume, deal with their emotional life, and exercise. They have a method of being active. They don't all run marathons, but they all move. They burn the calories either at home or in a gym. They put in the time, which can be as little as 30 minutes a day. Some have a trainer, but most work out alone. They usually do a variety of things that include strength training and cardio work. Some of them like group training, which is offered at many gyms.

Additionally, they develop a new mind-set about their manner of eating by realizing their health and longevity depend upon being in shape. People who get in good physical shape have more energy and feel considerably better about themselves.

Winners take the guess work out of what they eat. They know the healthy foods to eat and which to avoid. Screen your food and your portions. Be knowledgeable about what you are eating. Be careful to choose nutritious foods. One patient told me it is not a chore to eat correctly now. She said it's like learning to play an instrument. Once you practice, it comes naturally.

Winners are not the people who support fast food restaurants, but they do learn to find nutritious foods wherever they go. Try to avoid fast and prepackaged food and seek restaurants that are health-conscious. Know the importance of eating fruits and vegetables and staying away from unhealthy foods.

Winners do not use food to pacify themselves when under stress. They have good coping skills and seek resolutions to problems. They are not easily distracted from controlled eating when faced with a problem. "I don't mix my eating habits with the tensions of daily living," says Doris, a patient.

Winners are people we can learn a lot from because they have beaten the odds. Charles lost weight after discovering an allergy to dairy. He said: "I began eating in a healthy way because of an allergy to milk products. Now I know what I can eat and what to avoid to feel good. I find the longer I continue to eat what is best for me, the easier it is to continue doing so. If you practice what is healthy long enough, it becomes a habit. You don't even realize you are sticking to a plan." The allergy helped put Charles on the path to eating right, but you don't have to have allergies to follow suit — just use the advice in this book as the guide. Once you start eating fresh food, you will come to crave nutritious foods the same way you crave unhealthy sweets and comfort foods. The reverse happens as well. Once you get healthy food habits established, you may feel sick eating high-fat and high-sugar foods.

AM I SUCCEEDING?

Sometimes it's difficult to know if you're reaching your goals, especially if you try to use others as a yardstick for success. Each of us has different goals to reach because we are not all the same size or age, nor do we have the same temperament. Some of us have greater distances to travel to meet our objectives. So when we are trying to measure our gains, we have to use a personal measuring device. Some questions you might ask yourself are: Have I noticed any progress since I started on this particular program? Am I any more pleased with myself? Am I any healthier because of my efforts? Am I more selective in my choice of foods? Have I incorporated exercise into my daily life? Have I been consistent with my efforts to be successful? If I have strayed from my plan, did I get right back on track to eat healthy and exercise? Have I noticed benefits I didn't expect? If you are honest, you will be able to judge the progress of your efforts. You should celebrate any and all successes.

At some point, healthy habits become as natural to you as brushing your teeth. Pay attention to how you look and feel. People who get their weight under control feel proud about their eating habits. A patient, Cheryl, says she knows she is doing well by the selection of healthy foods she buys, as she now automatically passes the poor choices by.

Those poor choices will always be there, but it's important to keep moving forward. Each day and week can be a new start if we need it to be. Don't make your journey all about the scale. Hopefully the scale continues to move until you reach your goal, but the way your clothes are fitting, your measurements, or generally how you feel are all indicators that things are going well. And remember, life is like playing tennis — there is always another ball coming for you at which you get to take your best shot. Put your best effort into achieving all your goals.

CHAPTER 11

FINDING YOUR FOOTING WITH FOOD

As a person interested in your welfare, I want you to never settle for less than the best life you can achieve and not think you are limited to reach your goals. I have seen so many people who were defeated before they started because they had feelings of inadequacy or envisioned the task at hand to be monumental. I've helped people climb mountains of obstacles who have been quite surprised at their achievements. If food has been your obstacle, you can start right this second to control what you eat. Make this day the day that you get into the driver's seat and decide that no food goes into your mouth without your permission. Until you begin to eat in a healthy way automatically, I am requesting you be your personal guard to apply what you are learning about good eating habits. If desserts that are fattening appear in your home, you have to decide what to do. What action you take will tell you how serious you are about getting healthy and staying healthy.

We do not intend to take any pleasure away from you that is derived from eating; in fact, we want to enhance it. However, we don't want you to put all your eggs in one basket. You need to find alternate ways to feel good other than eating. This book offers you an improved lifestyle with a lot of healthy food choices. Keep an open mind if the choices are new to you. We bet you'll find you like your new way of eating better than what you have been used to.

An awful lot of my overweight patients would tell me they hardly eat. It is true that people vary in metabolic rates and some may gain weight even when eating lightly. But usually when folks are overweight, it is because they are eating too much food. One of my patients told me repeatedly that she hardly ate but continued to gain weight. When I asked her to keep track of what she consumed during the day, she was most surprised. Even with knowing she was going to write down whatever she ate, the long list was quite revealing. This means that a conscious effort is needed until you get into new habits. It takes thinking carefully about your food choices and the amount of food consumed to change. Without thinking carefully, we are prone to grab things at any time and eat throughout the day — and all of that snacking adds up.

My daughter's concept of eating for health and not for comfort is a great one. Healthy foods can protect our bodies from cancer and inflammation as well as provide immunity for us. Unhealthy foods make us sick and are leading to medical problems in incidences never seen before. Sometimes we derive so much happiness from eating that we forget there are other ways to seek pleasure. Those who overeat tend to associate eating with feeling good, a sense of fullness, and generally being happy. We have been programmed to use food for pleasure, comfort, and calming, and now we need to be deprogrammed. We've also become a food-obsessed country. So many people tell us that they think about food all the time. Thinking about your next meal or snack will interfere with a productive life. I witnessed thousands of my patients lose weight simply by focusing on improving the quality of their lives. I believe that when they were able to focus on being healthy, productive, and attractive, food became less of a focus and weight fell off.

FINDING NON-EDIBLE SOLUTIONS TO PROBLEMS

We know that people who are overweight use food as a comforting tool. They eat to make themselves feel better. That is their method of choice to gain satisfaction. There is a tremendous surge of adrenaline (excitement) and dopamine that occurs while eating candy, cookies, and ice cream. It's imperative that you learn new ways to cope other than eating. The next time you're faced with some trauma, avoid automatically going for the comfort foods. Make a list of all the things you do that make you happy or console you. Make a list of the people in your life who are helpful and positive. This way, you can call your favorite aunt or e-mail your college roommate for comfort instead of eating. Then make another list of new things you'd like to try. You will find that a busy schedule of seeking pleasure and fun will deter you from thinking about your next meal. Whether it's going on a photo safari in Africa or just drinking herbal tea while reading an inspirational book, the activities can be anything as long as they're not centered around food.

Find productive solutions to your problems; get help if you need it. Find new hobbies and interests. As an example of alternative ways to feel better, you may consider singing, joining a theater group, dancing, reading, making a photo album, learning to play a musical instrument, going for a walk, etc. The point is there are multiple ways to seek pleasure other than eating. Mike, a retired policeman, said he started overeating because his schedule was pretty empty. Once he got involved in a seniors group, he did not focus on food so much.

Food is tricky in that it's packed with connotations, memories, and emotions. It can also be just plain tasty. Foods that are especially loaded with salt, sugar, and fats can indeed be quite irresistible. No wonder we gravitate toward them and go overboard to seek them out. Tom told me he is hooked on pizza. Check out his comments: "I go to this pizza place, which is near my office. I like the place and they know me by now. What's the sense of my ordering a few slices? I know I'm not going to be satisfied. So I order a whole pie. Do I need the whole pie? I don't need you to tell me that it is not in my best interest. It's my habit." I told him we were at an impasse. He can't trim down and have his pizza, too. I asked him how he felt eating the entire pie. "I feel like a jerk. That's how I feel. I can't get into my clothes," he said. I was finally able to help Tom see that he was creating several problems for himself. He was making both his feelings of self-worth and weight problem worse. Maybe the next time you are questioning whether you should eat something, you might ask yourself if the given food will add to your self-esteem.

Sure, eating a pizza can feel great for a couple of minutes — but you are capable of much greater accomplishments than eating an entire pizza. Once you are closer to your goal weight, there is nothing wrong with enjoying pizza in moderation. Many people reading this book haven't proven to themselves that they can be successful. I want you to think of your road to successful eating as a new venture, a venture that can indeed be very exciting. Maybe you've never realized the benefits that come from concentrating on eating whole grains, more vegetables, and fruit. When you take out cake and candy from your diet, you will truly appreciate the sweetness of fresh fruit. Maybe you've never realized the impact of the fatty foods that have been messing up your arteries. Maybe you never gave much attention to eating a healthy breakfast.

Know that we are not taking anything away from you — we're only adding. There's an abundance of foods available that will add to your enjoyment. Think of a new plan of eating as going on a pleasant journey. Watch out for the inner messages you will be sending yourself. I want you to say to yourself: "I can lose weight and I am going to get healthy. Success is within my reach and I am going to make it happen."

Once your brain gets on board with your new eating habits and you're able to see food as fuel for nourishing your body — not the comforting friend that you've thought of it as, or the mindless indulgence you place into your mouth without thought — you'll have cleared the biggest hurdle toward the new, improved you. Once you have this attitude shift, food will change from destructive for you to protective for you.

CHAPTER 12

THE POWER OF EXERCISE

Losing weight is a marathon, not a sprint. My wife, Benita, is a 12-time marathon runner who's completed the 26.2 miles 11 times in New York and once in Dublin, Ireland. If she used up all her energy in the first few miles, she'd never be able to complete any of her races, let alone a dozen of them. She also didn't start running until her late 40s. I remember she had gained weight, and when she announced that she aspired to run a marathon, my four children and I were surprised. But she succeeded and is still exercising regularly at age 79. I often hear her and other runners talk about having a runner's high. Their running stimulates neurotransmitter activity, sending a wave of endorphins to the brain. Despite how grueling a race is, these runners associate exercise with pleasure, not with pain. You may not want to train for a marathon, but the word is out that the benefits from exercising are a vital part of being healthy. This is a component you must have, in some way, shape, or form, if you want to be successful for years to come. Benita is no longer running marathons, but she still exercises on a regular basis. Incidentally, training for a marathon takes time, as does reaching any sort of athletic goal. If you have a significant amount of weight to lose, be patient for it to drop off.

When it comes to working out, I frequently hear comments such as "I get enough exercise walking around at my job" or "it's boring" or "I don't believe it's necessary." These are all untrue. Try to identify those messages you send to yourself that are not in your best interest. Try to catch the excuses that will keep you from being successful at controlling your weight. Don't avoid stairs or walking short distances unless you have some compelling reason to. This might require breaking habits you've held for years, but it's all in your best interest.

If you didn't grow up knowing the importance of exercise, you're not alone. There was a time when bed rest was the preferred treatment when a patient had a heart attack or operation on the knee or hip. Now doctors know the benefit of getting patients moving soon after surgery. I recall when Dwight Eisenhower suffered a heart attack, those in the medical profession were surprised that his physician had him exercising soon after the operation. In the 1950s, the benefits of exercising were not so well known. Now we know better. Consider this: If exercising is so beneficial to many after an operation, imagine the benefit it can have to keep us all mobile.

Although more people are exercising today than in past years, there are still an overwhelming number of individuals who make excuses for living a sedentary lifestyle. When preparing to write this book, I made a habit of asking people why they do not exercise. Joe, who is considerably overweight, told me he had tried it a few times and did not notice a difference. He was not convinced that exercising is a lifelong activity needed to stay healthy, and his effort a few times was not strong enough to produce a habit. He brushed off the subject without acknowledging the importance of being physically active. Tim responded to my question by saying exercising is no fun. He is at least 75 pounds overweight. Some of the other excuses I heard were: "my schedule is too busy to exercise" and "I normally walk a lot when I have time" and "we have a gym where I work but dressing and undressing is too much of a hassle" and "I eat less instead of working out" and "I don't think it's worth the energy" and "it's not for me!" (with no explanation) and "I will when I have more time."

If any of the above sound familiar or you are coming up with your own excuse for not putting some form of physical fitness into your daily routine, you are deluding yourself into thinking you have a valid reason for excluding exercise from your life. One of my close friends is currently hampered by a knee injury that makes walking difficult. Nevertheless, she exercises frequently from a sitting position and walks with a walker. Let reading this section be your signal to *get moving*. Stop the excuses and stop waiting for more time in your schedule. Make the change now. Your health depends on it.

I recall reading about a General Bradley, who was a West Point graduate. When he was old and confined to a wheelchair, he was thinking about his life and how he faithfully exercised. He attributed his health and strength throughout his life to having made working out a priority. I think of that as I dependably go to the gym five times a week. I get a good feeling knowing I am doing all possible to stay in shape. I look in the mirror and feel proud of what I see. That is the way I would like you to feel. If you have any negative feelings regarding exercising, please get them out of your mind. You may feel so overweight you think you will be embarrassed, or you may not know where to start. You may feel you will be bigger than the people there. You may have a million reasons and excuses not to exercise. Whatever your reasons, stop the negative thinking and excuse making. You need to exercise to stay healthy and maintain the weight you lose, as well as reduce the stresses in your life. If you're at a public fitness facility, you can get help with using the equipment, and the other people will respect you for being there. You can also choose to exercise at home. Dr. Rebecca and her husband are both busy physicians who make exercise every morning at home before work a priority. My daughter prefers solitude when she's working out, and she enjoys exercise time as alone time. Find what works for you. I have personally always been more motivated to exercise at a gym, where there is a great deal more equipment. Also, the music, companionship of others, and the general ambience are conducive to exercising for me. When schedules are hectic, home exercise or walking outdoors may be easier to stick with. If it's quiet, it can also be a nice time for meditation, and all forms of exercise are great for reducing stress.

AVERTING A CRISIS

I asked a patient, Tony, what motivates him to attend the gym. "I am in the real estate business, and whenever anyone mentioned exercising, I would tell them I did plenty of walking showing space to clients," he said. "To tell you the truth, I never gave it too much thought. I always knew I was overweight, but it was something I accepted because I loved to eat and drink. My wife was always after me, but I felt that was normal. You asked me why I come to the gym and I am telling you everything but. What turned me around? I had a business partner. We had insurance policies on each other to protect the business. When we took them out, we thought we would live forever. Last year, my partner had a heart attack and died. He was 51 years old. We were about the same age and weight. I can't tell you why it took his death to get me into the gym, but it did. Since I've been going, I've lost a few pounds, but the real thing that motivates me is that I feel protected being here. I now go to my doctor on a regular basis, too. I feel like I have two important bases covered, and the odds are with me to live a healthy life. My partner dying was like getting a shot in the arm. Now that I am doing it, I can't figure out why more people don't exercise." That's a pretty powerful story. Hopefully you got the message not to wait until a crisis before doing what is healthy. This is particularly important if you fall into the obese or morbidly obese categories on the body mass index chart, as this is where catastrophes happen.

It is indeed an important message, as failure to exercise is responsible for an estimated 2 million deaths worldwide each year, according to the World Health Organization. That means that somewhere around 60 percent of the global population is not keeping up with the minimum recommendation of exercising 30 minutes a day. Health care costs continue to rise. Millions of Americans cannot afford insurance. Billions of dollars are spent annually in the United States on heart disease alone. If more people got the message to exercise, imagine the impact it would have on the health care industry.

Better yet, imagine the impact that exercise can have on you — unless you're not interested in looking better, feeling better, having more energy, and getting sick less often (just to name a few benefits), now is the time to find an exercise plan that works for you.

CHAPTER 13

GETTING YOUR LIFE IN ORDER

I want to prepare you for success in an area where many people fail. I have seen many people go all out to lose weight for a wedding or an important event that was coming up in their life. Right after the occasion, they gained all the weight back. I know when people feel confident and have good coping skills, they make permanent life changes. We all have that kind of exciting potential. Many don't reach their potential because they anticipate failure and rejection or throw other obstacles in their path to success. Losing weight is important but not the whole story. I want to help you truly be in command of your life and psychologically the best person you can be. The confident, self-reliant, goal-oriented person who seeks solutions to problems does not settle for mediocrity in any area of his or her life.

I, too, had to learn this lesson. When I went into private practice, I was ready to save the world. Nothing could stop me from seeing patients. Hardly any time was devoted to lunch or dinner. What I ate was consumed in haste between patients. Additionally, I worked long hours. I did play tennis and swim once in a while, but I had no regular plan to exercise. Dinner was at 9 or 10 p.m. when I got home from the office. A busy life can really throw a wrench in the works and prevent one from having an organized and healthy lifestyle. Take an inventory of your life to see if you're treating yourself well. You may be surprised at what you find.

"I WOULD LIKE MORE FOR MYSELF"

If you feel like you've been getting nowhere in your quest to get healthier, you may need to look at your life more holistically — are you emotionally where you want to be? My most memorable patient, Elsie, shed the extra weight she had gained once she got her life back on track. If she had only dealt with losing the excess pounds and not making herself well again in all areas of her life, I don't think she would have been successful in the long term. Here's her story:

I first saw Elsie when she was 18 and brought to my office by her parents. They were concerned because she was pregnant and wanted to marry the father of her baby. They did not think she, nor the boy, was ready for marriage. As I listened to Elsie's story, it was obvious that the idea to get married was hastened by the fact that a child was coming. Both she and her boyfriend had intended to go to college. We talked about giving the child up for adoption. Elsie did not want to consider that. We talked, too, about her relationship with her boyfriend, Peter. She thought she knew him well enough to build a lasting relationship. I got the impression that marriage was primarily her idea. She admitted that Peter would consider an abortion or giving the baby up for adoption. I attempted to get Elsie to continue to see me. I thought the matter to be too important to rush a marriage. She did not return for help. I later learned that the couple married.

The next time I saw Elsie was six years later. She had gained considerable weight. Her opening remark was: "I should have listened to you the last time I was here." I asked what had happened since the last time we met. "Peter and I married, but it was no good," she told me. "He didn't want to be with me. So we had the marriage annulled. I have a beautiful 6-year-old son, but he doesn't have a father. I have a decent job with the phone company but never went to college. Nothing has been ideal, but my parents really love my son."

"What brings you here today?" I asked.

"You may think I wasn't paying attention when my parents brought me here. I had a lot going on in my head. I knew Peter wasn't excited about getting married. I knew I wasn't going to give up my baby. And I knew I wasn't ready to take care of a child. I was feeling pretty stupid and my mind was closed. I knew you were trying to get me to sort things out. All my friends were going off to college and I was going to be a mother. Well, here I am six years out of high school, with a job that isn't challenging, trying to be both a mother and a father to my son, and terribly overweight. I would like more for myself and don't know how to make it happen."

It was obvious that Elsie was not proud of herself. The job with the phone company paid for her apartment and babysitters. She hadn't given up on the idea of being married but hadn't gone out socially for six years. We had a lot to talk about. Elsie had no specific goals in mind but wanted a more challenging career so that she would feel better about herself and be better able to support herself and her child in the event she did not marry. She didn't want to spend four years in college and still be undecided as to a vocation.

She decided nursing would appeal to her. Over the next three years, with the help of her parents, Elsie graduated from nursing school, lost considerable weight, and got married. Elsie had read my first book. When she called to tell me how well things were going, she asked how I was. I told her I was in the process of writing a book with my daughter. She kind of choked up and said, "Tell my story, Dr. Herman. See if you can help young girls avoid making some of the mistakes like I made." It wasn't easy for Elsie to get her life in order. She knew she would have a better lifestyle with a career in nursing. Her achievements as a nursing student gave her confidence in herself. Being in the hospital setting among people gave her the incentive to eat better and exercise. When she looked and felt better, she was more receptive to dating.

Everything was connected, and improving each aspect of her life got Elsie to all her goals. Going through my records to ascertain why some patients have been successful losing weight and keeping it off, I've noticed time and time again that those whose life is in order make the most progress. Maybe they resolved a personal problem. Maybe they got out of a stressful situation. Maybe their mood was elevated. In most cases they were feeling better, more relaxed, and had resolved a problem that was causing tension and unrest.

"THE PROBLEM WE HAVE GOES WAY BEYOND WEIGHT"

Another case stands out in my mind. A young lady named Frances came to see me about her husband, who was grossly overweight. She said she kept after him to lose weight, but he did nothing about it. She described him as being a nervous wreck and difficult to live with. She reported, too, that he had been to their family doctor and refused to stay on a diet. She asked if I would see him. Two weeks later, I received a call from Donald asking for an appointment. Here is what he said to me: "I don't know what Frances told you, but the problem we have goes way beyond a weight issue. Notice I said 'we.' I am not a stupid man and I know my weight is a problem for me. There was a time when I was in shape and ate more wisely. This weight has been building up in the past five years. I'm going to tell you the truth; otherwise, we are wasting time. I like my wife as a person, but I don't want to be married to her. We are like oil and water. She doesn't know that because she's in her own world. I haven't done anything about the situation because I can't think of where to start. There are the children, the finances, my job, her feelings. I came today thinking maybe you could sort things out. She is a good woman, but we are no good together. Can you help me?"

Donald continued to see me and was able to learn to cope with his personal problems. As he did, he began to take better care of himself, feel more relaxed, and lose weight. As you begin to choose more healthy foods to eat and exercise, pay particular attention to your feelings to determine if you have any unrest in your life that needs your attention. Are you relaxed or are you plagued with anxiety, depression, fears, guilt, or anger? When people have emotional strength and self-confidence, they are more prone to think and act better. Hopefully you will be able to learn something from Donald's story. His tale is about someone who needed a little assistance from a professional. Your tale may be able to be resolved by yourself. If you're not sure if you need help, discuss the matter with your physician.

"I DON'T KNOW WHAT TO DO"

A common time to need a little extra help is after a tragedy. That's when I first met Mary, who made an appointment to see me a month after her husband died suddenly at the age of 55.

Mary was left with three small children and a big restaurant they both operated. She was overwhelmed with grief and experienced feelings of helplessness wondering how she could cope with all she had to do. When I first saw her, she talked about the fear of breaking down emotionally, the business failing, and not being able to cope with her responsibilities. When she told me all she had achieved prior to her husband's death, I could tell she was a woman of many strengths but momentarily feeling swamped with duties that had been shared with her husband. As she calmed down and was thinking rationally, she decided it would be best to sell the restaurant. Once it was sold, she felt considerably better and could devote her attention to the children and thinking about her next moves. The new owners of the restaurant offered her a part-time position as a hostess, which she found a good break from her routine of caring for the children.

When Mary realized that her grief and helpless feelings were normal and temporary, she began to see her strengths and took pride in not only surviving the tragedy of her husband's death but emerging a strong and capable person. In the process of recuperating from the tragedy, she felt stronger, started taking better care of herself, and lost considerable weight. What we can learn from Mary's story is that there is a period of calm after the storm of a tragedy when one's strengths to cope come to the surface.

"I DIDN'T WANT TO SPEND MY LIFE ALONE"

Elsie, Donald, and Mary were pretty unhappy with the way their lives were progressing, but sometimes even when things seem to be going well for someone from an outside perspective, that person can be ready for — and need — a change on the inside. That happened with Doreen, a 29-year-old actress who had a theater career centered around playing the role of a heavyset woman. When she first came to see me, she told me that she may be ruining her opportunities to get parts in plays but was tired of being overweight. Here is what she had to say after losing 70 pounds: "I have always wanted to be an actress. I was in so many plays in high school and college, I was confident of acting professionally. I have done well but never liked being overweight. When I came to see you, I had made up my mind that my happiness was more important than my job. If I am as good an actress as I think, I should be a better actress now that I am thinner. My agent discouraged me from losing weight. I got rid of him. I feel terrific now. I am sleeping better and have more pep since I've been exercising. I will never let myself get out of control again. You asked me what made me decide to lose weight. I realized I had a lot of friends, but I wasn't a person who men looked at to date. I don't want to spend my life alone. I want to build a relationship with someone who sees me as attractive. You have to admit I look a whole lot better than when I first came in." It was like a bell had rung in Doreen's head signaling her to take action, and she certainly did.

LEADING A BETTER LIFE

Although we have written this book to primarily help you eat in a healthy manner and control your weight, we hope you will take a personal inventory to ascertain if all your thoughts and actions are in your best interest. We want you to be thrilled with who you are and with the life you are creating. For example, do you get enough sleep? There was a time when I made a lot of demands on myself to get up early and work late, thinking I was strong and could get along on five hours' sleep. I found out it is not so. I was tired in the middle of the day and needed a nap. We almost all need that seven or eight hours of rest to function at our best. There are many studies about seven hours of sleep being needed for weight loss. These days, I get into bed at 10 p.m. with a book and may read for a half hour before falling asleep. I wake up about 6 a.m. rested and eager to start the day. There are exceptions to that sleeping habit, but basically I stick to that rule.

Because I am a student of human behavior, it always interests me to inquire about a person's life. "Who are you?" I might ask someone. I like to know how people are traveling through life — what they do with their time, their occupation, their education, their family ties, and any other information they share is all interesting. I notice, too, whether someone smokes and if that person is in decent physical shape. When people smoke heavily or are considerably overweight, I worry about their self-control. If the conversation is friendly, I might ask questions. If I sense the person is receptive to change, I might offer my card and suggest he or she check out my personal growth book. If the person is defensive, there won't be much of a conversation. If, however, the individual is gregarious and likes the fact that I show interest, the conversation could lead to something meaningful. Just as I take an interest in those whom I meet, these words are my way of showing an interest in you. Each of us should be on the lookout for enhancing the quality of our life. Hopefully, you will be sparked to direct your thinking toward getting healthy and making other improvements in your life. If I am lucky, some of my copy just may ignite that flame to steer you to a more exciting life.

CHAPTER 14

THE TIME TO CHANGE IS NOW

The epidemic of obesity in the United States, the monumental marketing influences to get us to eat foods that are not in our best interest, and the cultural phenomenon to associate food with the height of pleasure have all placed people in a vulnerable position. The number of individuals at a dangerous weight is alarming, and you should never feel that you're alone. It is clear that many people would like to be in better health, gain approval from others, and derive positive feelings from being attractive and in good physical shape. That's exactly what you can do, starting now.

I make many observations about myself as I travel through life. One observation is that there are good days and better days. Never is there a bad day, because each day is a gift. As I spend time in the gym, I notice there are days when exercising is a breeze and all takes place effortlessly. There are other days when it seems to take more effort than usual. We change from day to day depending on our mood, how rested we are, how we are feeling, and what is on our mind in terms of unfinished or unresolved business.

You will also have good days and better days. We don't all react the same to the same plan because we vary in emotional and physical makeup. Metabolism and nutrient requirements can be different from one person to the next. Please be patient if it takes you a little longer to see results. If all doesn't go well with what you're doing, regroup and continue to try. Try not to find fault with yourself, but do continue to move forward, and consider professional help if you really feel stuck.

When I was writing my book *Secrets from the Sofa*, I considered a number of titles, including *Change Your Thinking, Change Your Life*; *The Road Map to Change*; and *Change Is Possible*. You've probably noticed the theme: *Change* is the operative word. It is what we all have to continually do if we want to live a dynamic life. If you at all care about living the best life possible, this is a great opportunity to make a change that you can be proud of. This is your big chance to demonstrate your inner strength and take charge of your life. The sky is the limit as to where your efforts will take you. It is a good idea to have goals. Present and future goals give us food for thought and something to look forward to. If you think about where you really want to go, you will get there.

You've probably spent a lot of time taking care of other people and things during your life, whether that be your kids, your partner, your parents, your career, or your community. You can do all that better if you just take care of yourself first. Anytime you get on an airplane, the flight crew will tell you that in case of emergency, you should put your air mask on first before assisting others. It's the same with taking care of your body.

It's amazing what we often put before our health. A patient of mine, Rolf, said he treated his car better than he did himself. "I was getting annoyed with myself when my clothes didn't fit and I was having difficulty getting through the day," he told me. "I was going to visit a customer and started talking to myself because I wasn't proud of the way I looked. All of a sudden it occurred to me that the car looks beautiful and I look a mess. I couldn't believe what I was seeing and feeling. How could I have neglected myself for so long?" Rolf woke up that day, made an appointment with his doctor, and is well on his way to becoming a person he can be proud of.

MY WISH FOR YOU

My life has been most productive, interesting, dynamic, and rewarding. I enjoy my relationship with people; the profession I have chosen; my role as a husband, parent, and grandparent; and the many activities that lend meaning to my world. I am grateful for the health and energy to continue on for as many years as possible. I like how I use my time. I like the way I look. I like the interests I've pursued, such as reading, lecturing, and being involved in charitable work.

What is that all supposed to mean? It all adds up to living a life you are proud of. I take care of myself and think and do the things that make me proud. That is the answer to taking charge of your life. You have an opportunity to get healthy. You have an opportunity to start being selective in what you eat. You have an opportunity to lose weight. If others can do it, so can you. It is not out of your reach. Just start and make it happen. Focus on it happening, not how long it will take. It's hard to think about your whole goal. Focus on the week ahead and the positive changes you are making. Focus on how meaningful the change will be in your life. Focus on how proud you will be to get control of your life. Don't make it complicated. Get excited about changing. When a patient tells my daughter that he or she will try to exercise or eat healthy foods, she says, "Don't try; just do it!"

Just as I am so pleased with the life I've created for myself, I want the best possible life for you, too. When you are 100 and you add up the years, I want you to be proud of all your efforts to live the greatest life possible. That's what every person deserves. Life is too precious to waste time not being at our best. Indeed, lost time is never found. Too many people do not get healthy and their lives are cut short. Losing weight adds years to your life. It may take the very serious, horrifying thought of leaving behind those you love to get you to change now.

The case studies throughout this book show that if you're committed to changing, patient, and ready to persevere, you can succeed. That's exactly what I want for you. Every person deserves the finest life possible. Yours starts today.

EAT **PLAN** MIND BODY

SECTION THREE

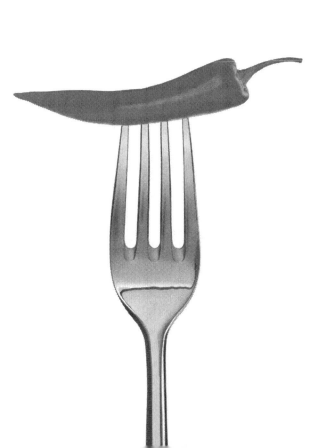

At this point, you are in the right mind-set to lose weight and know why you should do it. Now comes the fun part — putting what you've learned into practice. This section is chock-full of resources to help you do just that, from exercises to assess where you're starting from to the lowdown on how to get your eating habits, schedule, and exercise working for you instead of against you. Follow this formula, and you *will* lose weight the healthy way.

When you lose weight with prepackaged food programs like Jenny Craig or Nutrisystem, you eat prepackaged food for six months, lose 40 pounds, then start eating regular food again and gain 50 back. On this program, we start today with real food. I have so much success with weight loss because we start with real food, and once we find healthy foods you like and a schedule of eating and exercise that works, weight vanishes. The transition is made in the beginning, so there is no adjustment back to real food as seen with other programs.

CHAPTER 15

A FORMULA TO GET STARTED

First, you need to make an accurate assessment of where you are with your weight and where you would like to be.

I like using the body mass index chart (see the Additional Resources section in the back of the book) because it is a general indicator of health widely used by doctors and nutritionists.

I am always trying to get patients to a BMI between 20 and 24 because that's the range where there is no increased risk of any medical problems. A BMI of 25 to 29 is considered overweight and comes with an increased risk of hypertension and diabetes, among other medical problems. A BMI of 30 or more is obese and holds the same medical risks as if you fall into the overweight category, plus heart disease; cancer; knee, back, and joint problems; and sleep apnea. A BMI over 35 is known as morbid obesity (in other words, obesity associated with death), and the risks include all the risks in the obese category, plus heart attack, stroke, and sudden death. If you are in the range of having a BMI of 30 or higher, your potential for medical problems is greatly increased and your life expectancy is shorter.

Please make an appointment with your primary care doctor prior to starting a diet and exercise routine to make sure you are healthy enough to start a program.

To assess your situation at this point, I'd like you to do two exercises. The first is to identify where you are currently and where you would like to be. Think of a weight you were happy with in the past and how you felt at that weight. Find a picture of yourself at that weight and put it up where you can see it every day. Don't worry if you have not been at that weight for years. Get as close to a BMI of 24 as you can for your goal weight.

Then write down your:
A. Current weight and current body mass index
B. Goal weight and goal body mass index
C. Current chest, waist, and hip measurements in inches

Write down your goal weight on pieces of paper and put them up around your house. Seeing this weight, possibly with a picture of yourself that you are proud of, all around your home will help it become a reality. Visualize yourself at that weight before you go to bed and when you get up in the morning. Spend at least 10 minutes doing this each day. Once you see yourself at this healthy weight, it will become your new reality. Make small goals if it will help you. In the office, we like to break up the ultimate goal with little goals. For example, if someone is 221 pounds during a weigh-in, I might set the goal for next week at 219 and a two-week goal at 215. When these numbers are broken down into smaller chunks, they seem more achievable.

Take measurements of your chest, waist, and hips periodically. In our office, we do this at three-month intervals. This will keep you motivated even when it seems like the scale isn't moving as quickly as you would like it to. Don't worry too much about the scale; weighing yourself once a week is enough. As long as you are moving in the right direction, be proud of yourself.

Exercise 2 focuses on current food and exercise habits. Write down what you normally eat on a typical day. Please include the snacks and times of all eating as well as any exercise you are currently doing. Don't worry if you can't accurately remember foods and times, because most patients who come to our center write the words "varies" or "all throughout the day" on their intake forms. Just do your best to recall what you've eaten, and don't gloss over anything — it's important to have a realistic view of where you're starting. Also, don't fret if your exercise is a big zero at this juncture. You cannot feel bad about your start point. This is wasted energy. The most important thing is that you are committed to improving your health. Losing weight and getting healthy is all part of a long journey, not a short race.

Activity	Time	On a typical day…
Breakfast		
Snack		
Lunch		
Snack		
Dinner		
Snack		
Exercise		

THE CHANGES START NOW

I am now going to give you a formula to analyze your life and weight loss troubles in the same manner I would if you were sitting in front of me in my office. You must take your current food choices and pull out bad fats and refined sugars. Some things may be obvious to you, like candy or cookies, and others may be more difficult to see. I want you to eliminate all white flour from your diet. This includes white bread, white rice, and white pasta. They have very little nutritional value and are linked with diabetes. All bread, pasta, rice, and cereal will be used sparingly until you get closer to your goal weight. I have tried this a number of different ways, and experience shows that if I give patients one-fifth a cup of rice or pasta, they tend to eat more of that food than is recommended, so it's best to cut it out entirely until later. I want you to succeed, and I find that our program average of three or so pounds a week is highly motivating. If you are able to take to these new habits and be serious and strict with yourself, you will see the pounds start to peel off. If you need to move slower with food elimination, this if fine because it is a step in the right direction — just remember that the results will be slower as well.

FOOD CHOICES

Take a good, hard look at the foods you eat most days. See if you can come to healthy choices for three meals and two snacks that will combine some protein with an antioxidant-filled fruit or vegetable at every meal and every snack. My favorite choices for breakfast are oatmeal with berries, an egg-white omelet with vegetables, or a high-protein cereal with berries. For the morning snack, I love a fruit and a nut or nut butter (all-natural peanut butter or almond butter). For example, an apple with one to two handfuls of almonds or walnuts, or an apple with 1 to 2 tablespoons of peanut butter or almond butter.

For lunch, I recommend either a big salad or soup and a smaller salad. Try to get some protein with your salad. It can have chicken, but the better choices still are nuts, beans, and fish. It's important to have one big salad a day. If you do this regularly, you'll begin to crave salad. Favorite afternoon snacks are cut-up vegetables and bean dip such as hummus or white or black bean dip. Favorite dinners are lean proteins (like fish) grilled or sautéed, a cooked vegetable, a side salad if you did not have one for lunch, or a side of beans and fresh fruit for dessert. If you have three meals and two snacks, you should not be hungry throughout the day or later at night.

It shouldn't matter if you are home or eating out. Good choices can be found anywhere if you're motivated to succeed. Please don't be afraid to ask at restaurants how items are prepared or what comes with certain dishes. For example, if chicken is fried, ask to have it grilled, baked, poached, or sautéed. If an entree comes with pasta, ask for a side of vegetables instead. You will be in control of what you order and still maintaining your healthy choices. Try to avoid frozen and prepackaged meals. This is usually accomplished by staying on the periphery of the grocery store. Frozen and packaged meals tend to have a higher amount of preservatives and are filled with omega-6 fatty acids that are linked with the chronic medical problems we are trying to avoid.

Drinking water should be part of every meal and snack. Try a lemon or lime slice in water or seltzer, but please avoid all regular and diet sodas. Regular soda has as much sugar as a piece of cake, and research has shown that diet soda is linked to everything from strokes and kidney problems to a larger waist circumference and fat formation around vital organs. Also, the artificial sweeteners in them can make you want more to eat. Natural is always better. Your great-great-grandparents did not face the obesity problems we have today, and beverage choices are a big part of it. You would not water your flowers with soda or give anything to your pets to drink but water. Treat your body the same way.

SCHEDULE

Now it's time to analyze your schedule. Are you skipping meals? If you are, give yourself permission to make time for meals. You'll only need a few extra minutes and the difference you'll see will be enormous. Please don't allow yourself to say, "I'm not hungry in the morning." If you are not happy with your weight and what you're currently doing isn't working, then change it. It will not happen overnight, but all the small changes are cumulative. I strongly recommend eating within an hour to an hour and a half of waking. Don't wait until you get to work to eat. By the time you get to work, it will be too late for breakfast and you'll be thinking about work and not about good food choices. I have helped thousands of patients by pushing their first meal closer to waking. I cannot stress this enough.

Try another exercise. This time, divide your day into times (be precise) for three meals and two snacks. This is the schedule you should adhere to as closely as possible. A typical day might include breakfast at 6:30 a.m., a morning snack at 9:30 a.m., lunch at 12:30 p.m., an afternoon snack at 3:30 p.m., and dinner at 6:30 p.m. — that's all the food for the day.

When you're eating, slow down and remember my Dr. Rebecca 18-minute rule, in which you take at least 18 minutes to eat because that's how long it takes your brain to process the fullness. Be mindful of what you're eating. Put your fork down in between bites and chew your food thoroughly. Partition your day and analyze what your bad times are. For many, it's the afternoon. If that's the case for you, start a scheduled snack at 3 or 3:30; don't wait until you're starving. If you get too hungry, that's when poor choices are made and large portions are consumed. Other common bad times are nights, weekends, or when eating out. Plan for these, and learn to analyze if you are really hungry or if you're eating just because you're in the habit of doing it. Many people snack while watching television at night. This is a great example of mindless instead of mindful eating. Replace that habit with something positive like drinking water or herbal tea during television time or while reading in the evening.

If you know you're going to be dining at a restaurant at night, eat the rest of the day as you normally would so you're not starved by the time you get there. Too many people make the mistake of not eating all day when they know they have a dinner out or an affair like a wedding. If you skip a meal, you will make it up later. Try to look at the menu ahead of time so you know what you'll order and won't have the extra pressure of searching for something healthy on the spot. Most restaurants have their menus online. If you have a plan for the day with eating, you will be less likely to overeat. (There are more tips for ordering out in a restaurant in Section 4.)

EXERCISE HABIT

Find one 30-minute block of time every day to do some cardiovascular activity that you enjoy, then make it happen. No excuses. This habit must be nonnegotiable. This is definitely the key to maintaining weight loss, yet so many people are unable to commit to it. Find your inner athlete and start thinking of this time as your "me time." You are never too old or too out of shape to start. One half hour is not a very big chunk of your day. Go to a gym if you like gyms or walk outside. Don't let yourself make excuses of being too busy or not a morning person. Everyone can change, and it doesn't matter where you go or what exercise you do — what matters is making the commitment to yourself to maintain exercise as a priority in your life. I always do at least one half hour of cardio a day first thing in the morning. This is true on a work day, a weekend day, a vacation day, or any other day. This is the kind of consistency it takes to maintain a healthy weight, and it's worth it for all the benefits exercise provides.

JOURNAL

Make a journal of your days going forward. (For a template to follow, see a sample journal in the Additional Resources section.) Include food choices, times, exercise, and mood. We learn so much about our patients by reviewing the week's journal entries, particularly in regard to foods eaten and exercise. Then analyze your own journal once a week. How many times did you exercise? How many healthy meals did you have? Did you skip meals? Did you have any days that you were unable to follow the program? If so, do you need to change your schedule? We are constantly tweaking the programs of our patients on a weekly basis. Do you need to move a snack earlier or later? Did your work schedule change? If so, readjust. You can always contact our center at www.popweightloss.com if you need help. We Skype weigh-ins with people in all geographic locations who need help. We can even make a program for you.

WEIGH IN

Try to weigh yourself once a week. There is too much natural variation in your body to weigh in every day, and weighing yourself too often can lead to discouragement. The weekly weigh-in, which should be done at the same time every week, if possible, will keep you motivated for the long haul. Don't be upset if progress is slow at first. Some people can grab all the new habits at once and some are slower. Too many people give up too soon. Stay with it because it will get easier day by day.

WEIGHT LOSS MEDICATION

I do use some FDA-approved weight loss medications if needed. These medications can decrease your appetite by up to 60 percent. I find that this can help decrease cravings and jump-start weight loss for some people. However, no medicine is magic. You must change your food, schedule, and exercise habits to have success. Also, these medicines need to be prescribed and monitored in a doctor's office.

Don't wait to get started — you will love the way you look and feel! If you start these exercises now, you will begin your journey today. My patients say I'm ruthless, but I do not like excuses. There is always a reason to wait and start later or tell yourself that next month will be better for you. There is always a season, holiday, birthday, or vacation coming up to use as an excuse to postpone starting. Respect yourself enough to follow these suggestions fully and start now. This is where you will see real results.

CHAPTER 16

THE FACTS AND FICTION OF FATS

To make good eating choices, it's helpful to know what the building blocks of food really are. This includes fats, which get a bad rap, but some fats are a necessary part of our diet, helping us stay full longer, keeping our skin healthy, and promoting the proper distribution of vitamins throughout our body. The key is knowing what food sources provide the kind of fat we want, as well as how much of that we should be getting — and what fats we need to avoid under all circumstances.

In his book *Good Calories, Bad Calories*, Gary Taubes explains that the idea "fat is bad, carbohydrate is good" has caused many problems for our country. Consumers decreased the fat in their diet but greatly increased the sugar, and that's helped no one. Just reducing the fat in your diet is not enough to improve your health. Cutting out fats is not the answer, but becoming more educated about them is.

So what's the difference between a "bad" fat and a "good" one? Let's start with the bad. Saturated fats, which are not good for you, are found in animal products, full-fat dairy, and some tropical oils. Saturated fat is solid at room temperature, like butter. Some of these fats have been shown to increase the risk of coronary artery disease, diabetes, and obesity.

Trans fats, another type of bad fat, are fats made from hydrogenated or partially hydrogenated vegetable oils and are found in margarine, vegetable shortening, commercial pastries, deep-fried foods, and prepackaged snacks. Trans fats make us store fat in our bodies instead of burning it. Like saturated fats, trans fats have been shown to negatively affect your health and are most likely even worse for you than saturated fat is. This is due to the fact that they're known to raise cholesterol.

Now for the kind of fats your body needs: Monounsaturated fats and polyunsaturated fats are usually derived from plants and are liquids at room temperature. Focus on replacing saturated and trans fats with monounsaturated and polyunsaturated fats, and the benefits will include a reduction in heart disease. This will mean a diet with fat sources from mostly fatty fishes, nuts, and seeds.

Monounsaturated fats can be found in almonds and avocados. These lower cholesterol, lower blood pressure, and positively affect health. Changing your thinking to increase the amount of monounsaturated fat in your diet is a great goal. With any fat, it's important to pay attention to portions. I always tell my patients to have one to two handfuls of almonds, not 17 handfuls.

Polyunsaturated fats are found in corn, safflower, and peanut oils. Polyunsaturated fats cannot be made in our bodies and must come from the food we eat. During digestion, the body breaks down fats into fatty acids, which can be absorbed in the blood.

OMEGA FATTY ACIDS

Under the polyunsaturated fats umbrella are two types of essential fatty acids to know: omega-3 and omega-6. Although they are related, they differ from each other because of their chemical structure.

Omega-3 fatty acids are found in seafood, mainly from the fat of cold-water fish such as salmon, herring, cod, mackerel, and bluefish. Omega-3 fatty acids are also found in vegetable oils like olive oil and canola oil, as well as walnuts and flaxseeds. They can be found in dark green leafy vegetables, legumes, and some herbs such as mustard fennel and cumin. The two forms of omega-3 that our bodies need are eicosapentaenoic acid, or EPA, and docosahexaenoic acid, or DHA. These are the building blocks for the hormones that control cell immunity and cell growth.

It's estimated that one-quarter of Americans eat no fish at all. This is so hard to believe, because the omega-3s in fish are protective for you. Fish consumption is shown to lower rates of dementia, improve cardiovascular and eye health, and increase life expectancy. According to the Environmental Protection Agency, concerns that fish is dangerous because of mercury levels and PCBs (polychlorinated biphenyls), synthetic compounds found in industrial and commercial waste, have been overblown and fish is largely safe to eat. Beef, pork, and chicken actually have higher dietary levels of PCBs and toxins. To be on the safest side, consume a variety of fish types. Also, the selenium present in most fish has a protective role against mercury. As long as fish is higher in selenium than mercury, there is no reason to limit to 12 ounces per week and it is safe to eat. Pregnant and breast-feeding women should eat two to three servings of cold-water fish per week.

The coronary heart disease benefits of only 6 ounces of wild salmon per week (250 milligrams/day) include fewer coronary heart disease deaths and a lifetime cancer risk reduction of 75 percent. In a study called "Fish intake, contaminants and human health: Evaluating the risks and benefits," published in *The Journal of the American Medical Association (JAMA)* in 2006, the authors noted that the Japanese population eats on average 900 milligrams a day of EPA and DHA, and has death rates from heart disease at 87 percent lower than in the United States. There is also evidence that fish consumption leads to a decrease in inflammatory and autoimmune processes.

The anti-inflammatory properties in omega-3s help us fight and prevent infection and should be a strong presence in our diets. They have *incredible* health benefits of lowering cholesterol, lowering blood pressure, and reducing inflammation. Omega-3 fatty acids have also been shown to prevent skin from wrinkling and elevate mood.

A 2002 study published in *JAMA* found that eating fish at least once a month can reduce the risk of ischemic stroke in men, while in a University of Pittsburgh study, Dr. Cyrus Ragi showed increased fish consumption seems to be protective against Alzheimer's disease. Numerous other studies have found a benefit to eating fatty fish, including one published in *Preventive Medicine* that showed that fish consumption was associated with a reduced risk from all-cause, ischemic heart disease and stroke mortality across 36 countries.

The second essential fatty acid is omega-6. This is found in vegetable oils like corn, safflower, and sunflower and in foods fried in these oils, or salad dressings, margarine, or mayonnaise made from these oils. It can also be found in chicken, olives, sunflower seeds, and pine nuts. Here, the primary fatty acids are linoleic acid and arachidonic acid. These fatty acids are not beneficial to our bodies. They tend to cause inflammation and most likely contribute to chronic medical conditions like heart disease and diabetes. While we need omega-6 fatty acids to function, the ratio of omega-3s to omega-6s should be improved.

The Lyon Diet Heart Study demonstrated that a good balance of omega-6s to omega-3s is 4 to 1, but some American diets now have a ratio as high as 20 to 1. This imbalance can lead to coronary artery disease, cancer, diabetes, asthma, arthritis, lupus, depression, and Alzheimer's disease.

SEVEN SIMPLE RULES FOR FATS

Don't try to eliminate fat from your diet completely, but do try to be smarter about what fats you eat. Here are some quick rules to follow:

1. Cut down on butters and use olive and canola oils sparingly. The fats from whole foods such as nuts and seeds have more beneficial properties than oils and will help you feel fuller longer.
2. Eat low-fat or part-skim dairy.
3. Steer clear of hydrogenated oils found in prepackaged pastries, prepackaged snacks, and fried foods.
4. Cut away visible fat on your meats and fatty skins on your fish.
5. Eat more baked and broiled fish; avoid fish that's fried. Focus on cold-water fish like salmon, sardines, herring, and anchovies that have the heart-healthy omega-3s. If you don't like fish, try some new ways to prepare it or at least supplement with 1200 kilograms of omega-3 fatty acids per day.

6. Get healthy nuts and seeds like walnuts, almonds, and sunflower seeds into your diet in moderation.
7. Work on improving your ratio of omega-3s to omega-6s.

Bad Fats, Good Fats

BAD FATS

What: Saturated fats and trans fats

Where: Red meat, full-fat dairy, butter, ice cream, hydrogenated vegetable oils, packaged baked goods

Why: Increases risk of chronic disease

GOOD FATS

What: Monounsaturated fats and polyunsaturated fats

Where: Nuts, seeds, cold-water fish, and some oils (in moderation)

Why: Decreases risk of problems such as diabetes, cancer, and high cholesterol

CHAPTER 17

CARBOHYDRATES MADE SIMPLE

Just as with fats, there's a lot of misinformation out there about carbohydrates. I think many people are addicted to carbohydrates. They're linked with emotional eating more than any other nutrient type. This can be a real addiction, but unlike nicotine or other addictions, we cannot live without food. What we can do is make better choices and work not to be controlled by sugary sweets. With 68 percent of American adults and up to 40 percent of American children overweight or obese, a diet overhaul is greatly needed in this country, and I think carbohydrates (sugars and starches) are our biggest problem. When we began to focus on low-fat foods, we unknowingly started eating foods higher in carbohydrates and got collectively fatter. We need to stop focusing on sugary foods for comfort and start making food choices for health.

Carbohydrates come in the form of sugars (such as fructose, glucose, and lactose) and starches (vegetables, grains, rice, breads, and cereals). The body turns most carbohydrates into glucose, a type of sugar, which is then absorbed into the bloodstream. This triggers the pancreas to release insulin, a hormone that moves sugar from the blood into the cells, where it can be used as a source of energy.

When it comes to understanding carbohydrates, it's important to learn the difference between simple and complex carbohydrates. Simple carbohydrates are made of one or two sugar molecules. They are digested quickly. They are fast energy sources and raise our blood sugar rapidly. They are found in candy, table sugar, white flour, maple syrup, and honey.

Complex carbohydrates are made up of long chains of sugar molecules that digest slowly. They have more fiber and keep blood sugars stable and are healthier for us. Complex carbohydrates are found in green vegetables, beans, lentils, peas, oatmeal, and foods that are made of 100 percent whole grains, such as brown rice and brown pasta.

I would like to point out that whole-food carbohydrates from fruits and vegetables, nuts, and beans are carbohydrates and are beneficial to our bodies. The carbohydrates from bread, pasta, and rice in the form of whole grains have nutritional value and should be incorporated once we achieve a healthy weight.

Simple carbohydrates have no bulk or fiber, so they do not fill you. Americans get far too many calories from white bread, pasta, rice, and sweets, and this directly leads to type 2, or adult-onset, diabetes. Diets high in refined and simple sugars cause our pancreas to release a surge of insulin. If that process is repeated over and over again, diabetes can result.

It's also important to eliminate artificial sweeteners. There is evidence that even no-calorie sweeteners increase cravings and increase portion sizes.

A *BERRY* GOOD CHOICE

Brightly colored fruits and vegetables are always great choices because they contain phytonutrients. Phytonutrients have anti-inflammation and antioxidant (anti-cancer) properties. Berries in particular have a tremendous amount of antioxidants, which are naturally occurring molecules found primarily in fruits and vegetables that protect your body's cells from damage caused by free radicals. There is evidence that cells damaged by free radicals are the cause of many cancers and chronic illnesses. This is why a diet full of fruits and vegetables can fight and may even prevent cancers. Berries are also low on the glycemic index, which is the rate at which a particular food raises your blood sugar. Blueberries have been shown to increase brain function, while blackberries are excellent for prostate health. Strawberries have recently been linked to lowering throat cancers and in their freeze-dried form contain even more antioxidant properties.

All fruits are not created equal, though. Bananas and raisins are near the top of the glycemic index and should be avoided for the most part until you are closer to your goal weight. You cannot think of these restraints as forever because they are not. It was hard for me to have any fruits restricted. I enjoy bananas at my goal weight now and have an average of half a banana twice a week. But it's important to eat all foods in moderation.

If you want to see results that promote motivation, be strict with the program. If fast results aren't important, then don't restrict any fruits or vegetables, but *do* get used to making healthier choices.

REGULATING BLOOD SUGAR LEVELS

The incidence of type 2 diabetes has skyrocketed in this country, and I believe this is largely due to refined sugars. Bleaching flours and bread to a white color essentially strips food of almost all its nutritional value. White bread has almost no fiber and acts like sugar in our bloodstream. The refining process is done primarily for shelf-life extension.

If you want to avoid diabetes, it's best to stay away from white rice, white bread, white pasta, white potatoes, French fries, soda, candy, and processed foods.

Whole-grain bread, pasta, and rice should be used sparingly until you reach your goal weight. Try to look for the words "whole wheat" and "100 percent whole grain" because sometimes foods are dyed brown but are not whole grain.

Low-glycemic foods release and raise blood glucose, or sugar, levels more gradually and are therefore better for you. These foods include legumes, or beans. Beans are very much underused in this country and I am always trying to get my patients to eat more.

The take-home message is that fruits, vegetables, nuts, and beans are carbohydrates, too, and focusing on them versus bread, pasta, rice, and crackers is a much better choice for you. I promise it will make a huge difference and is likely to keep you from diabetes and other health problems.

In general, all white flours, breads, pastas, rice, and baked goods (especially prepackaged ones) have a very high glycemic index, while vegetables and fruits, nuts, and beans have a low glycemic index and are better choices. White potatoes are my main exception to this rule and should be avoided until you are closer to your goal weight.

Wondering how foods rank on the glycemic index? Here are some examples. The lower the number (on a scale from 1 to 100), the less the food affects blood sugar and insulin levels.

Food	Glycemic Index
Baguette	95
White rice	89
Soda crackers	74
Watermelon	72
Raisins	64
Hamburger bun	61
All-Bran cereal	55
Oatmeal	55
Green peas	51
Potato chips	51
Brown rice	50
Orange juice, unsweetened	50
Macaroni	47
Pear	38
Tomato juice	38
Carrots	35
Skim milk	32
Black beans	30
Wheat tortilla	30
Pearled barley	28
Grapefruit	25
Peanuts	7
Hummus	6

Source: "International tables of glycemic index and glycemic load values: 2008" by Fiona S. Atkinson, Kaye Foster-Powell, and Jennie C. Brand-Miller, December 2008 issue of Diabetes Care

SIMPLE RULES OF THE DAY FOR CARBOHYDRATES

1. Eat three servings of fruit each day. Make one serving a cup of berries. Servings can be one regular-sized fruit or one cup of berries or cut melon.
2. Eat at least four serving of vegetables a day. I make vegetables unlimited on my program. Try to get in vegetables that have high antioxidant and anti-inflammatory properties. (See a list of these in the Additional Resources section.) Swap all of your crackers and pitas for fresh vegetables.
3. Have one big salad a day.
4. Have a quarter cup of beans per day.
5. Replace dessert with fresh fruit.
6. Get rid of artificial sweeteners.
7. Get rid of all sweetened beverages and opt for water.
8. Look at the "Total Carbohydrate" section of food labels — the lower the number, the better. Most foods you choose should have 10 to 15 grams per serving at most.

Antioxidant Cheat Sheet

Here are some of the basic antioxidants and how they help our bodies. Most of the benefits are derived from getting your antioxidants from fruits and vegetables and not from supplementation.

Beta-carotene is found in sweet potatoes, cantaloupe, carrots, and fruits with orange and yellow colors. Beta-carotene can be converted to vitamin A, which helps protect bones and vision.

Lycopene, found in red fruits and vegetables, is a powerful antioxidant for our skin and can reduce your risk of skin cancer. Lycopene has also been shown to be protective for the heart, eyes, and prostate. The best sources of lycopene are tomatoes, watermelon, and red peppers.

Flavonoids are found in berries; green, white, and black tea; onions; herbs; and spices. Flavonoids fight aging and prevent disease.

Ascorbic acid, also known as vitamin C, is found in citrus fruits, berries, papayas, and dark green vegetables like spinach and broccoli. It is needed to form collagen in bones and muscles.

Vitamin E is found in nuts and nut butters, avocados, eggs, green vegetables, and whole grains. Vitamin E protects body tissue from damage and helps our immune system fight viruses and bacteria.

Selenium helps regulate the thyroid and immune system and is in fish like mackerel, tuna, halibut, flounder, herring, and smelts; shellfish like oysters, scallops, and lobster; garlic; whole grains; and sunflower seeds.

CHAPTER 18

PROTEIN SOURCES

The nice thing about protein — the third essential energy source for the human body — is that if you're eating a balanced diet, you don't have to worry much about whether you're getting enough. That's good, considering that protein is needed for building tissue, making hormones, and transporting oxygen through the blood, just to name a few functions.

While people often think that meat is the best source of protein — every vegetarian is inevitably asked, "But how are you getting your protein?" — that's not the case at all. Yes, meat does contain protein, but there's protein in most vegetables, and likely more than you think. In his book *Eat to Live*, Dr. Joel Fuhrman asks what has more protein: broccoli or steak? If you guessed steak, you are wrong. Steak has 6.4 grams per 100 calories and broccoli has 11.2! Dr. Fuhrman also points out that even romaine lettuce has more protein than steak — but without the saturated fat.

Nuts, seeds, and beans have the great quality of providing protein along with the properties of the "good" fats. They are also so easy to prepare that they can be eaten just about anywhere. I think a good principle and an easy way of adding this to your day is to focus on nuts, seeds, and beans as part of a salad for one meal of the day. By doing this, you will feel full but not too full, and portion sizes will not get too large. Also, you will get the added benefits from the variety of vegetables and fiber in your salad. These plant proteins lower cholesterol and decrease the incidence of heart attacks.

While a plant-based diet is often the healthiest, going completely vegetarian or vegan is so much of a change that it's unrealistic for most. Also, many of my patients come in adopting a diet with no meat and dairy, but they replace those lost food groups with too much bread, pasta, and rice. These individuals become nutritionally deficient, lacking essential omega-3 fatty acids and many of the benefits from fresh fruits and vegetables, nuts, and beans. If you don't want to go entirely meat- or dairy-free, focus on having one meal a day with fish, chicken, beef, or dairy, and one meal that is vegetarian for your lunch and dinner.

If you have any chronic diseases or really want to make a major change, you might want to consider trying out a vegan diet. Animal proteins have no fiber and no antioxidants (or anti-cancer properties) and are in fact linked with chronic lifestyle diseases such as heart disease, diabetes, and cancer. This is also true with dairy, even low-fat dairy. Dr. Dean Ornish, author of *Spectrum*, says that the Asian diet of fruits, vegetables, legumes, whole grains, soy in its raw form, and fish used as a condiment can reverse heart disease and cancer. If you struggle with many medical problems, especially high cholesterol, hypertension, and diabetes, you should consider a balanced vegan diet. It will most likely reverse your medical conditions. Americans have far too many animal proteins in their diet, despite long-term evidence of the detriments. A 1993 study published in *The Journal of the American Medical Association* called "Body weight and mortality:

A 27-year follow-up of middle-aged men" showed those who avoided meat and dairy had lower incidences of heart disease, blood pressure problems, cancer, diabetes, and obesity.

If you do eat meat, consider that over-cooking, as in barbecue, has been shown to be carcinogenic (cancer causing). Whether it's on a nut or a hamburger, the blackened color from over-cooking should be avoided.

We always joke at Pop Weight Loss that we operate a "chicken clinic" because the amount of people who eat chicken for lunch and chicken or turkey for dinner is far too great. I feel some of our nutritional problems in this country stem from this lack of variety and the inability of people to try new things. We are always asking our patients to keep an open mind. By this I mean break out of patterns of eating that are not working for you and think in terms of your health. This is easier to do if you keep in mind that fruits and vegetables, nuts, and beans will give you the most nutritional value and the most immunity for your body.

Step outside of your regular patterns and search for proteins from sources like vegetables, legumes, nuts, and seeds. Try to minimize large quantities of animal proteins. Look at the protein you choose for fiber content and nutrient value. I have always liked the concept of using protein, especially meat proteins, for flavor or as a condiment — that might mean having a salad with a few small pieces of chicken or a little shredded meat in a soup, as opposed to having the meat at the center of the plate.

Remember that replacing meat with processed white flours like crackers, rice cakes, and pretzels will do nothing for you nutritionally and will most likely cause you to gain weight. It is the large amount of unprocessed plant foods that give us immunity for disease. Eating a diet rich in fruits and vegetables and using meat and dairy sparingly, while adding nuts, seeds, and beans for protein to your diet, is the best way to go.

CHAPTER 19

THE SKINNY ON SUPPLEMENTS

Nobody is perfect; we all can use some help when it comes to getting the nutrients we need. I am often asked whether I feel vitamin and mineral supplementation is beneficial. Although my overall philosophy includes eating many fresh fruits and vegetables, nuts, and beans, with some fish and animal protein as a condiment, I do think supplements have value.

The key, however, is to think of them as exactly that — supplements. They are an aid to a good diet, not a replacement for eating well. They cannot turn poor habits into good ones.

So what should you be taking? Your personal doctor is the best person to help you come up with a plan tailored to you, but here are some things to consider:

A high-quality **multivitamin** gives us some leeway with our diet. I caution against megavitamins for many reasons. Megavitamins that contain high amounts of vitamins A, E, and D are not water soluble and can build up in your system. This could be very serious if, for example, you were pregnant and didn't know it. The effects of these vitamins as well as high amounts of beta-carotene and folic acid may be harmful to us and should not be taken in doses higher than the recommended daily allowance unless prescribed by your doctor.

Vitamin D deficiency is becoming more common. Getting a blood test is smart. If the level is normal, 800 IUs of vitamin D is a recommended maintenance dose.

Calcium supplementation for women over 45 years old is 1200 milligrams per day, taken in divided doses. It can help protect bones, along with regular exercise. A diet rich in calcium is thought to improve blood pressure. Even though dairy is a good source of calcium, people are always surprised to learn that many fruits and vegetables like oranges, broccoli, and tomatoes are rich in calcium as well.

Omega-3 fatty acids, or DHA, are recommended as a 1200-milligram supplement. This should be taken in addition to eating omega-3-rich foods, such as green leafy vegetables, cold-water salmon, walnuts, and flaxseeds.

Chromium picolinate is the precursor to insulin and metformin, which are medicines used to treat diabetes. Chromium in addition to low-sugar foods and eating on a healthy schedule can be helpful for stabilizing blood sugars throughout the day. The usual dose is 100 to 200 milligrams twice a day.

5-hydroxytryptophan is a sleep aid that I sometimes use with patients. Tryptophan is the substance in turkey that makes you tired and it also has an appetite suppressant. I like to have patients take this with dinner or before bed to decrease nighttime eating. Please do not take this supplement if you are taking an antidepressant and do not drive after taking it.

A good nonprescription aid is green tea and coffee extract combined with raspberry ketone and mango extract. This combination is thought to increase total weight loss by up to 10 percent by decreasing appetite. At our Pop program, we have a supplement that includes these substances called **Pop Boost**.

I am a proponent of **probiotics**. Probiotics are digestive microbes that decrease the inflammation in your colon and help with normal bowel habits. I recommend them if you have to take antibiotics or you have any bloating and constipation issues. There are also toothpastes made with probiotics, which may be helpful if you struggle with many dental or gum problems.

Remember, please check with your doctor before starting any supplement regimen.

EAT

PLAN MIND BODY

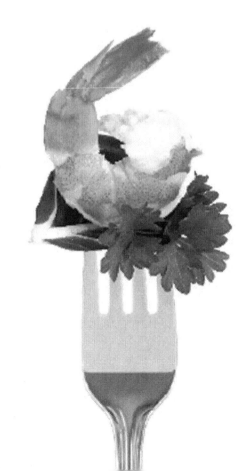

At the heart of any (good) weight loss effort is a plan for eating. Of the three pillars of Pop — food, schedule, and exercise — food is often the most difficult for people to make adjustments to. While all three are needed to lose weight, maintain that loss, and stay healthy, making good food decisions plays a huge role in getting to the weight you want to be. There are so many choices with food that it can be overwhelming figuring out what the smartest options are. This section gives you concrete ideas on what you can eat for all meals and snacks, as well as how to shop for food, prepare it in your home, and order it when you're out.

CHAPTER 20

WEIGHT REDUCTION INDUCTION PHASE

When you're first starting out with the plan, it may seem like a big adjustment, but it will soon become a lifestyle change that you'll want to keep up. Eat protein (4 ounces lean poultry, fish, beef, dairy, or beans, or 1 to 2 ounces of nuts or nut butter) with a serving of vegetables or a serving of fruit for meals. (Oatmeal or a high-protein cereal may be used as protein for breakfast. See the food selections and sample meals that follow.) All vegetables may be consumed during induction except corn, carrots, white potatoes, and beets. All fruits may be consumed except bananas, raisins, cranberries (fresh or dried), and mangoes. All foods should be grilled, steamed, baked, or sautéed.

Eat three meals and two snacks a day. Do not skip meals, but you can skip a snack if you are not hungry. Try to eat slowly and enjoy your food. Try to get used to 30 minutes for meals and 20 minutes for snacks. Try not to eat after 7 p.m. Use protein in combination with fruits and vegetables for every snack and meal.

No bread, pasta, or rice during the induction phase. Grains such as oatmeal or cereal are acceptable for breakfast. Whole grains will be introduced in the maintenance phase. Focus on whole-food carbohydrates, which are fruits, vegetables, nuts, and beans.

Limit dairy during the induction phase because dairy can cause bloating. You may have low-fat dairy three times per week during induction, with more frequency during the maintenance phase. If you have no problems tolerating dairy, or you have increased blood pressure (dairy has been shown to have an effect on lowering blood pressure), you may consider more dairy.

Drink plenty of water. Drink 8 ounces of water before each meal and snack. Try to drink a minimum of ten 8-ounce servings of water per day. Mineral water or seltzer with lime or lemon is acceptable. You may drink iced unsweetened green or black tea, but remember that any drink with caffeine can be dehydrating, so for every coffee or tea consumed, please drink two glasses of water. Try to wean from all diet sodas and drinks with artificial sweeteners.

Exercise at least 30 minutes every day. If you are not sweating, you are not working hard enough. People who combine a healthy diet with exercise lose more weight and maintain the weight they lose. Find your time to exercise and make it nonnegotiable.

A multivitamin with at least 800 milligrams of vitamin D and 1200 milligrams of omega-3 fatty acid plus a probiotic is recommended for weight loss and maintenance.

CHAPTER 21

HOW TO SHOP

Please shop one to two times per week — but avoid it when you're hungry. Steer clear of the middle aisles in most supermarkets, which is where the junk food resides. You need fresh fruits and vegetables to achieve success; be sure to select the fruits and vegetables in season at the time. Wash and cut them up, then store in the refrigerator so they're readily accessible for snacks and meals. Use see-through containers so you don't forget about them.

Here's what to look for when you're shopping:

PROTEINS

Acceptable Meat Choices

Portion: 4 to 6 ounces for meals (4 ounces for most women and 5 to 6 ounces for most men); 1 to 2 ounces for snacks, or 1/4 cup to 1/2 cup for snacks

Lean beef, lamb, pork, veal, chicken (skinless breasts or thighs), turkey, Canadian bacon, turkey bacon, hamburger (90% lean or greater), chicken or turkey sausage, sliced roast beef; choose lean cuts, cut away visible fat, and do not eat the skin (yet cooking with it will improve taste)

Acceptable Meat Alternative Choices

Portion: 4 to 5 ounces for meals; 1 to 2 ounces for snacks, or 1/4 cup to 1/2 cup for snacks

All bean burgers including soy (try to make your burgers by using tofu, but packaged versions are acceptable), vegetable burgers, or Portobello mushrooms
Pop Protein Shakes (high in protein, gluten-free, and vegetarian): 1 scoop for meals, 1/2 scoop for snacks

Acceptable Fish Choices

Portion: 4 to 6 ounces for meals or 1 cup for fish salads; 1 to 2 ounces or 1/4 to 1/2 cup for snacks for fish salads

Cold water preferred; branzino, canned low-sodium tuna, catfish, clams, cod, crab, Dover sole, flounder, grouper, halibut, lobster, mackerel, mussels, oysters, salmon, sardines (packed in water), sashimi, scallops, sea bass, shrimp, snapper, tilapia, tuna

Acceptable Bean Choices

Portion: 1 cup for meals; 1 ounce or 1/4 cup for snacks

Black beans, cannellini, chickpeas (or garbanzo beans), edamame, hummus, kidney beans, lentils, navy beans, tofu, white beans

DAIRY

Acceptable Dairy Choices

Portion: 3 ounces or 1 cup for meals; 1 ounce or 1/4 cup for snacks; limit yogurt and cottage cheese to three times a week

Cheeses: all nonfat or low-fat cheese (cheddar, farmer's, blue, mozzarella, and feta are options), 3 ounces per serving
Cottage Cheese: low-fat or 1% or part-skim or nonfat ricotta
Eggs: regular eggs (limit to 4 per week if using yolks); may have 1 hard-boiled egg for snack
Egg Whites: 3 to 4 egg whites or egg substitute
Milk: 1% or skim milk; 1% or skim soy milk; Skim Plus; almond milk (only in cereal or drinks)
Yogurt: 1 cup nonfat plain Greek yogurt (higher in protein) or nonfat plain yogurt, but any low-fat or part-skim dairy is acceptable

FRUITS

Acceptable Fruit Choices

Portion: 1 cup of berries or cut-up melon; 1 small fruit; 1/2 for large fruits; limit to three times a day

Apples, unsweetened no-sugar-added applesauce, avocado, blackberries, blueberries, cantaloupe, cherries, grapes, grapefruit, kiwi, lemon, lime, nectarine, peach, pear, 1/2 orange, 1/4 cup pineapple, plum, raspberries, strawberries, cantaloupe, honeydew, watermelon

Avoid raisins, bananas, cranberries (fresh or dried), mangoes, and canned fruit until maintenance phase or closer to desired weight; frozen fruits are acceptable if you are unable to do frequent shopping

GRAINS

Acceptable Grain Choices

Portion: 1 cup; limit to three times a week

Cereal: Oatmeal, Cheerios, All-Bran, no-sugar Kashi cereals, or Hi-Lo (organic brand)

VEGETABLES

Acceptable Vegetable Choices

Portion: vegetables are unlimited

Artichokes, asparagus, green beans, broccoli, bok choy, Brussels sprouts, cabbage, cauliflower, celery, cucumber, dill pickles, eggplant, kale, leeks, lettuce, mushrooms, onions, peppers, radishes, scallions, shallots, snow peas, spinach, tomato, turnip, zucchini

Avoid carrots, corn, peas, white potatoes, beets, and canned vegetables until maintenance phase or closer to desired weight

FATS

Acceptable Fats Choices

Portion: 1 ounce or handful of nuts or olives; 1 to 2 tablespoons olive or canola oil; 1 to 2 tablespoons no-sugar-added or all-natural peanut butter or almond butter; 1/4 avocado

Raw or roasted (no salt) almonds, cashews, walnuts, peanuts, pecans, olive oil, canola oil, sesame oil, black olives, sunflower seeds

DRESSINGS/BONUS FOODS

Portion: 1 to 2 tablespoons

Olive or canola oil; low-fat and low-carb dressings with less than 2 grams of fat, sugar, and total carbohydrates; light mayonnaise or mayonnaise made with olive oil; red wine vinegar; white or apple cider vinegar; mustard; low-sugar ketchup; lime or lemon juice; all spices; garlic; low-sodium soy sauce; Tabasco; horseradish; wasabi; cinnamon

DRINKS

Water, mineral water, seltzer, coffee, tea (decaf preferred), unsweetened iced tea
Try to wean yourself off all diet drinks, and try to wean from all artificial sweeteners

Limit sugarless gum to two pieces per day; having too many pieces causes bloating

CHAPTER 22

FOOD PREPARATION GUIDE, BY COURSE

I have a confession to make: I'm not a good cook. You don't have to be, either (but if you are, all the better!). Unlike me, my husband is a terrific cook. He has the type of kitchen mind that can re-create barbecue sauce if we are out of it because he knows what's in there. Over the years, he's taught me many tricks for preparing food and making it tastier.

I've put these ideas into this guide in an effort to pass them onto you. Over the years as I've sat with weight loss patients, I've noticed that the most problematic mealtime is dinner. Many people feel that work, children, and time constraints mean they cannot stick to healthy eating. This doesn't have to be the case. I find that if you make a rough plan for the week, even if that means getting takeout two days and eating out twice, you will be able to execute a weekly dinner plan and not feel the pressure and panic at 7 p.m. that your only option is pizza or fast food. The goal of this section is to provide you with a realistic food guide. I aim to give you quick and easy ideas for meals and snacks that you'll be able to prepare on a regular basis.

Start with a menu for a week that fits with your schedule. Decide on a structure that works for your family and commitments, and then you can fill it in. For example, if you will need to bring in takeout on Tuesdays, make a schedule including Chinese takeout on that day and do a rotation of steamed shrimp and snow peas, or steamed chicken and broccoli. Make it fun and easy to plan — something like Meatless Monday, Fish Friday, and Steak Salad Saturday can become family traditions and help you plan and shop for the week. Try using a slow cooker or Crockpot, which can help you have a meal ready when you walk in the door. Double up any recipes that can be frozen for additional meals, such as soup and chili. Breakfast foods for dinner with vegetables or smoked salmon omelets are always a quick option.

The following will help you plan dinners, along with all other meals:

DRINKS

I'm starting the guide with drinks, an overlooked but very important part of any food plan. Protein drinks or yogurt smoothies can be used for quick snacks and meals. Try to vary what you put into them so you can get freshness and variety into your day. We are a nation that is on the go, and as much as I resisted offering shakes initially (finding the perfect one took some time), our patients enjoy the convenience of our shakes, which are made from a high-quality whey protein that is gluten-free and vegetarian.

BASIC POP PROTEIN SHAKE

1 scoop Pop Protein for a meal; 1/2 scoop for a snack
1 to 1 1/2 cups of water or low-fat milk
Up to 1 cup fresh or frozen fruit (no sugar added)
Ice

CHOCOLATE PEANUT BUTTER SHAKE

1 scoop Pop Protein in Creamy Chocolate
1 to 1 1/2 cups of water or low-fat milk
1 tablespoon natural peanut butter
Ice

RASPBERRY SHAKE

1 scoop Pop Protein in Creamy Vanilla or Creamy Chocolate
1 to 1 1/2 cups of water or low-fat milk
1/2 cup raspberries (frozen or fresh)
1/2 cup frozen rhubarb
Ice

CHOCOLATE COFFEE SHAKE

1 scoop Pop Protein in Creamy Chocolate
1 to 1 1/2 cups of water or low-fat milk
1/4 cup almonds, peanuts, or cashews (optional)
1/4 cup fruit (optional)
1 to 2 teaspoons instant decaffeinated coffee (may also substitute
flavored coffee, coffee extract, or espresso powder)
Ice

ALMOND CHOCOLATE NUT SHAKE

1 scoop Pop Protein in Creamy Chocolate
1 to 1 1/2 cups of water or low-fat milk
1 tablespoon almond butter
1/2 teaspoon cinnamon
1/2 cup fruit (optional)
Ice

YOGURT SMOOTHIE

(This can be made with yogurt alone or together with Basic Pop Protein Shake)
1 scoop Pop Protein
1/2 to 1 cup plain or Greek reduced-fat yogurt (nonfat Greek yogurt is thickest)
1/4 cup fruit (optional)
Ice
Reduced-fat milk or water if needed

DIPS

Three dips I love to use as snacks with raw vegetables or sauces for main courses are hummus, guacamole, and salsa.

Make your own or look for prepared brands that have less than 10 grams total carbohydrates per serving. This should be about 1/4 cup at the most for sauces and dips.

Hummus is made from chickpeas (also called garbanzo beans), tahini (a sesame seed paste), garlic, sesame oil, and lemon.

Guacamole is made with avocado, tomato, onion, olive oil, and lemon or lime juice. It is very filling and can be used as a snack with raw vegetables, as part of a salad, or as a side. Also think of avocado slices on sandwiches or burgers, or cut up in your favorite soup or salad.

Salsa is made from fresh chopped tomatoes, garlic, onion, lime juice, and cilantro. Fresh salsa is so much better nutritionally than ketchup; try it over scrambled eggs, as a condiment with burgers, or as a topping for fish. I have been successful in getting many patients to try fish by putting a fresh salsa or marinara sauce on it.

Find your own favorite dip combinations by experimenting. Puree cannellini beans with reduced-fat cheese and fresh herbs. Combine black beans with low-fat Mexican white cheese. Certain cheeses and herbs match well together, like basil and tomato with low-fat mozzarella, or sage with low-fat cheddar. Another example is goat cheese with fresh chives (especially good in an omelet). If you find a combination that you really like, you will be more inclined to stick with it for the long haul.

SALADS

Living by the one-big-salad-a-day mantra is a great way to get fresh vegetables and the phytochemicals you need into your diet. I like the idea of one big salad for lunch. Salads are a great way to experiment with nonmeat options. Quick and easy salads can be made with lettuce such as romaine, arugula, spinach, green, and red leaf. Adding nuts such as almonds, cashews, and pecans can add protein, as can seeds like sunflower seeds. Adding small amounts of firm tofu, fish, chicken, and steak can easily provide variation so you don't feel like you're eating the same thing day after day. It's a chance to think of fish and meat as a condiment or flavor rather than as the main focus of the meal. My suggestion is to find foods you already enjoy and put them over salad. If you enjoy them, you will stick with eating them once you achieve your goal weight, and then the concept of diet food is over. Use the food you make for the week by putting leftovers such as salmon or roast chicken in salads. Make extra exclusively for this purpose.

You can add light or olive oil mayo to your leftovers with celery to make all sorts of salads. I like to put a little mustard into my chicken or salmon salad and then make lettuce wraps from them. Add your favorite reduced-fat cheese for variety. I like reduced-fat crumbled blue cheese with steak salad, and reduced-fat Gorgonzola and sliced pear over mixed greens. Sometimes I add chicken for variety. Firm tofu cut into small cubes over lettuce with grilled vegetables and low-sodium soy sauce for the dressing is filling and very healthy. Many restaurants are doing interesting salads these days, so if you're stuck for ideas, get inspiration from their menus and re-create the salads you like (and make them healthier, if necessary) at home. If you're bringing your salad to work, try using containers with built-in compartments so your lunch stays fresh.

For dressing, I recommend making your own vinaigrette. Try combining red wine, white wine, or champagne vinegar in a ratio of one part vinegar to three parts olive oil. To this oil and vinegar base, you could add mustard, dried or fresh herbs, garlic, or lime or lemon.

If you're on the go and there is not a prepared salad, look for cheese and vegetables, hard-boiled eggs and fruit, or tuna or chicken salad. Try to omit the crackers, pita, and croutons. A plain grilled chicken salad or fresh deli turkey can be found most places, as can a plain Greek yogurt with fresh fruit.

SOUPS

Soups are great for lunch or dinner. Lentil soup is filling, and having it with a salad for lunch will not leave you feeling sluggish in the afternoon. Many patients feel so much better after eating soup and salad for lunch and abandoning old habits of sandwiches and pizza. Chili is also a nice choice and will leave you feeling full but not tired. Try different combinations, but make sure to have some protein either in your soup or your salad. If I have a vegetable soup, I make sure to put nuts or beans in my salad. If you are making soups from scratch, make extra and freeze in individual portions for later.

VEGETABLES

Vegetables are amazing for your health, providing anti-cancer and anti-inflammation properties that we all need. Getting more vegetables into your diet is the main objective. Try putting vegetables in a shallow roasting pan, drizzle with olive oil, and add salt and pepper or a spice for variety and bake for about 20 minutes. This can work with Parmesan cheese sprinkled over vegetables as well. This is my daughter's favorite way to enjoy asparagus. Ideas for vegetables include spaghetti squash to replace pasta and cauliflower mixed with ricotta cheese to achieve the texture of mashed potatoes. Vegetables used as main dishes that are flavorful and filling include grilled Portobello mushrooms and eggplant casserole. Placing chopped vegetables on a skewer over a grill pan or barbecue is another idea.

MAIN COURSES

CHICKEN

I try to get my patients to think about alternate proteins because it seems that chicken and turkey make up the majority of American dinners. Still, chicken is a good choice in moderation. My tips for dinner include making a few flavorful dishes well and then expanding from there. When you cook chicken on the bone rather than cooking up a skinless, boneless breast, it is much more flavorful. A quick foolproof way to make more-flavorful chicken breasts is by placing tinfoil over a shallow roasting pan. Rub the chicken breast with olive oil, salt, and pepper and bake at 400 degrees for 45 minutes.

A roast chicken is easy to make and can be used for dinner and lunches to follow. Buy a 6- to 8-pound chicken, take the insides out, and rinse thoroughly with cold water inside and out and pat dry. Take a lemon and whole clove of garlic, cut in half, and put it in the bird's cavity with herbs such as sage and rosemary. Then tie the legs together with string and tuck the wings underneath the bird. Place in a roasting pan and rub the outside of the bird with salt, pepper, and olive oil. Bake for about an hour at 425 degrees until the juices run clear. Take it out of the oven, cover it with tinfoil, and let it rest for at least 15 minutes. This recipe will get you through a special meal or any weeknight dinner.

FLANK STEAK

I recommend eating red meat no more than once a week. Flank steak is very simple to make and can be used for lunches in steak salads. It's important to take a flank steak out of the package and let it come to room temperature for 15 minutes. Unlike chicken, do not wash steak, but do salt and pepper both sides to taste. Preheat the oven to 350 degrees and place 1 to 2 tablespoons of olive oil in a hot, ovenproof pan (do not use nonstick), put in the flank steak, and leave it alone for about 5 minutes. Using tongs, flip the steak and place it in the oven for about 20 minutes. Carefully take the steak out with a glove and cover. Place the pan back onto the stovetop. Deglaze the pan with chicken or beef stock and add 1 teaspoon of brandy or sherry. Let the pan reduce by half and use as a gravy. Cut the flank steak perpendicular to the grain on the meat. I like this with mushrooms and other vegetables.

FISH

I try to eat fish at least three times a week and recommend this to my patients, too. Fish is easy to order at a restaurant and can be prepared at home as well. Baking fish in a tinfoil pouch is simple and makes cleanup easy. This recipe works with any fleshy fish such as salmon, halibut, and cod. Take a quarter-size sheet pan and cover it with two sheets of tinfoil. Take a fish fillet between 4 to 6 ounces skin side down or skinless and put 1 teaspoon of olive oil under and on top of the fish. Give a squeeze of fresh lemon juice and any fresh herb like parsley or a dry herb like thyme, and salt and pepper to taste. Fold your tinfoil into a pouch and bake at 350 degrees for about 20 minutes until the fish is cooked to your liking.

For thinner fish like flounder, grouper, or sole, I like to sauté in olive oil and sometimes add a very small amount of butter. With the skin side down, leave in the pan about 4 to 5 minutes and then turn the fish over for usually 1 minute. Take the fish out of the pan and put the juice of 1 lemon or lime into the pan to use like a sauce. You can also try coating the fish with mustard when done or put 1/2 a lemon and 2 tablespoons mustard off the heat and put it on top of the fish.

If you are not in the habit of cooking fish at home, try soaking fish in a little salt and lime prior to cooking it. Then sauté onions, shallots, garlic, and olive oil. With the known anti-inflammatory properties of onion and garlic, this can be the base start of any sauté. Then add sage, turmeric, or a small amount of clove, cumin, or paprika. Place your fish in, add water to cover the fish, and simmer until fish is cooked. This combination takes the fishy taste out, and by changing the spice, you can change the flavor dramatically.

Clams, mussels, and shrimp all make great appetizers in a restaurant in a small portion, or as a main dish. I prefer white wine sauce over a marinara sauce, but both are acceptable.

BURGERS

Burgers are quick and easy and can be made from many healthy sources, such as tofu, beef, poultry, fish, or Portobello mushrooms. Add a whole-grain bun for children or when you are at or close to your goal weight. Burgers are great over salad, or with small patties, as a side dish. I like adding a fresh fruit or vegetable salsa, guacamole, or hummus. Make one night of the week burger night.

DESSERTS

For desserts, it is imperative to think about fruit. The natural sugar in most fruits is wonderfully sweet and perfect for dessert. Many variations, such as freezing blueberries or baking apples with cinnamon, are superior to any candy to me. Also, cocoa powder can provide a delicious taste (with really no extra calories or carbohydrates) to foods such as nuts.

Berries with cinnamon or nutmeg are delicious and can be served alone or as a sauce over other fruits. I often ask for berries or fresh fruit for dessert in restaurants even if I don't see it on the menu. I also have my rule at home with my daughter that if she is hungry after dinner, she can only have fruits and nuts.

Fruit with part-skim ricotta cheese is also a wonderful option for a snack or dessert. Baked, grilled, or warm fruits with part-skim ricotta cheese are delicious and simple to make. Adding 1 teaspoon of vanilla extract can enhance flavor.

Apple, pear, plum, or peach slices with cinnamon or nutmeg are my favorite desserts. Slice thin, sprinkle with cinnamon, and bake 400 degrees for 1 hour.

Substituting cocoa powder for chocolate and adding black beans to brownie recipes can provide sweetness but keep you on a healthy diet.

SPECIAL-OCCASION TIPS

The average American consumes approximately 2,000 calories at Thanksgiving and holiday meals.

- Do not go to Thanksgiving dinner or any special occasion hungry. Eat breakfast and lunch as if it were a normal day. If you start dinner without eating all day, you will overeat.
- When making your plate, don't overdo it. Divide your plate into sections: one section for vegetables, one section for meat or fish, and another section for salad. You can always have a second serving of vegetables or salad.
- Drink a lot of water; it will keep you hydrated and help you not to overeat.
- Don't forget to slow down and enjoy your food. If 20 minutes have passed and you are feeling full, stop eating. Try to eat only until you are 80 percent satiated; eating too much will only make you feel sick and emotionally out of control.

BARBECUE TIPS

- Grill vegetables and fruits, place them on skewers, and make kabobs.
- Grill lean chicken, steak, hamburgers, and fish and vegetable burgers. Trim any fat before barbecuing the meat or fish.
- Have burgers without the bun and put them over a salad.
- Have chicken without the skin.
- Avoid potato salad and macaroni salad.
- Avoid any fried foods, bread, and rice dishes.
- If you're unsure of what foods will be there, offer to bring something you know you can eat.

CHAPTER 23

SAMPLE MENUS AND MEAL IDEAS

These three weeks of sample menus should give you a good idea of what you can eat during the day to be both healthy and satisfied. Dessert is always optional.

MONDAY

Breakfast: Pop Protein Shake with 1 cup berries and skim or 1% milk
Snack: Apple with 24 almonds (raw or roasted)
Lunch: Spinach salad with cucumbers, radishes, and tomatoes with 4 ounces grilled chicken (olive oil and red wine vinegar)
Snack: Celery with 1/4 cup hummus
Dinner: 6 ounces salmon with asparagus
Dessert: Fruit

TUESDAY

Breakfast: 1 cup plain oatmeal with 1 cup berries
Snack: Peach with low-fat string cheese
Lunch: 6 ounces tuna fish with 1 tablespoon light mayo over arugula salad
Snack: Celery with 2 tablespoons all-natural peanut butter
Dinner: Halibut with bok choy
Dessert: Fruit

WEDNESDAY

Breakfast: Egg-white omelet with spinach and tomatoes
Snack: Apple with 2 tablespoons all-natural peanut butter
Lunch: Chef salad with olive oil and red wine vinegar
Snack: 1/2 cup Greek yogurt (plain 0% fat) with pineapple
Dinner: Edamame burger with Brussels sprouts
Dessert: Fruit

THURSDAY

Breakfast: 1 cup Greek yogurt (plain 0% fat) with 1 cup berries
Snack: Pear and 20 pecans (raw or roasted)
Lunch: Asian salad with cabbage and romaine hearts with 6 ounces grilled shrimp (olive oil and red wine vinegar)
Snack: Cucumbers with 1/4 cup tzatziki sauce
Dinner: Chicken burger over cooked spinach with butternut squash fries
Dessert: Fruit

FRIDAY

Breakfast: Pop Protein Shake with 1 cup berries and unsweetened soy milk
Snack: Peach with low-fat string cheese
Lunch: Egg-white omelet with peppers and onions
Snack: Celery with 2 tablespoons almond butter
Dinner: Shrimp cakes with broccoli and cauliflower
Dessert: Fruit

SATURDAY

Breakfast: Egg-white omelet with vegetables and 2 pieces turkey bacon
Snack: Apple with 20 cashews (raw or roasted)
Lunch: Lettuce wraps with 4 to 5 ounces low-sodium turkey (deli meat)
Snack: Cucumbers with 1/4 cup hummus
Dinner: 4 to 5 ounces flounder with broccoli rabe
Dessert: Fruit

SUNDAY

Breakfast: Pop Protein Shake with 1 cup berries and skim or 1% milk
Snack: 1/2 cup Greek yogurt (plain 0% fat) with fruit
Lunch: Salad with 1 cup chickpeas, red onions, and string beans (olive oil and red wine vinegar)
Snack: Celery and peppers with 1/4 cup guacamole
Dinner: Scallops and grilled zucchini
Dessert: Fruit

MONDAY

Breakfast: Pop Protein Shake with 1 cup berries and skim or 1% milk
Snack: Fruit with 24 almonds (raw or roasted)
Lunch: Lettuce wraps with 6 ounces tuna fish and 1 tablespoon light mayo
Snack: Hard-boiled egg with kale chips
Dinner: Portobello mushroom burger with steamed string beans
Dessert: Fruit

TUESDAY

Breakfast: 1 cup Greek yogurt (plain 0% fat) with 1 cup berries
Snack: Apple with 2 tablespoons all-natural peanut butter
Lunch: Egg whites with broccoli, mushrooms, and spinach, plus a salad
Snack: Celery with 1/4 cup hummus
Dinner: Vegetarian chili and hearts of palm
Dessert: Fruit

WEDNESDAY

Breakfast: 1 cup oatmeal with 1 cup berries
Snack: Celery with 2 tablespoons almond butter
Lunch: 1 cup Greek yogurt (plain 0% fat) with 1 cup fruit
Snack: 2 ounces turkey slices rolled with lettuce and mustard
Dinner: Grilled shrimp with mixed grilled vegetables and a side salad
Dessert: Fruit

THURSDAY

Breakfast: Eggs in a muffin tin and 1 cup fruit
Snack: 1/2 cup part-skim ricotta cheese with fruit
Lunch: Grilled salmon watercress salad (olive oil and red wine vinegar)
Snack: Butternut squash chips with 24 almonds (raw or roasted)
Dinner: Lentil soup with cauliflower and side salad
Dessert: Fruit

FRIDAY

Breakfast: Oatmeal with 1 cup fruit
Snack: Apple with almonds (raw or roasted)
Lunch: Roasted chickpeas over salad with cucumbers and tomatoes (olive oil and red wine vinegar)
Snack: Celery and cucumbers with black bean dip
Dinner: Baked mustard lime chicken over sautéed spinach with garlic
Dessert: Fruit

SATURDAY

Breakfast: Eggs with mixed vegetables and 1 cup fruit
Snack: Apple with 2 tablespoons all-natural peanut butter
Lunch: Spinach salad with sunflower seeds and tomatoes
Snack: Hard-boiled egg with raw peppers
Dinner: Tilapia with salsa and snap peas
Dessert: Fruit

SUNDAY

Breakfast: Egg-white omelet with mixed vegetables and 1 cup fruit
Snack: Apple with 24 nuts of choice (raw or roasted)
Lunch: Roasted chicken with grilled asparagus
Snack: Celery with 1/4 cup guacamole
Dinner: Tofu vegetable stir-fry (or protein of choice) with a side salad
Dessert: Fruit

MONDAY

Breakfast: Oatmeal with cinnamon and 1 cup berries
Snack: Apple with 2 tablespoons all-natural peanut butter
Lunch: 6 ounces tuna with 1 tablespoon light mayo stuffed in pepper
Snack: Kale chips with tzatziki sauce
Dinner: 4 ounces filet mignon with grilled zucchini
Dessert: Fruit

TUESDAY

Breakfast: Pop Protein Shake with 1 cup berries and 1% or skim milk
Snack: Hard-boiled egg with fruit
Lunch: Cauliflower pizza with kale salad
Snack: 1/4 cup roasted chickpeas with cucumbers
Dinner: Tofu burger with grilled eggplant
Dessert: Fruit

WEDNESDAY

Breakfast: Egg-white omelet with 1 piece of Canadian bacon
Snack: 1/2 cup Greek yogurt (plain 0% fat) with 1/2 cup berries
Lunch: Cannellini beans with kale and salad
Snack: Trail mix (1/4 cup high-protein cereal and 1/4 cup favorite roasted nuts) with fruit
Dinner: Pork and pineapple with cabbage slaw
Dessert: Fruit

THURSDAY

Breakfast: Egg-white omelet with asparagus
Snack: Fruit with low-fat cheese
Lunch: Egg salad (2 eggs) with 1 tablespoon light mayo over bed of red leaf lettuce
Snack: Butternut squash chips with 20 pecans
Dinner: Garbanzo bean burger with cooked spinach
Dessert: Fruit

FRIDAY

Breakfast: 3/4 cup part-skim ricotta cheese with 1 cup berries and skim or 1% milk
Snack: Celery and any nut butter (1 to 2 tablespoons)
Lunch: Lentil soup and salad
Snack: Muffin in a cup
Dinner: Stuffed peppers with sautéed mushrooms
Dessert: Fruit

SATURDAY

Breakfast: Egg-white omelet with mushrooms
Snack: Raw vegetables with 1 cup hummus
Lunch: Greek salad with 4 to 5 ounces grilled chicken (olive oil and red wine vinegar)
Snack: Fruit with pumpkin seeds
Dinner: 1 cup bean salad with steamed Brussels sprouts
Dessert: Fruit

SUNDAY

Breakfast: Egg-white omelet with spinach
Snack: 1/2 cup nonfat cottage cheese with fruit
Lunch: Turkey chili (add mustard greens/kale) with tomato salad
Snack: Peppers and cucumbers with 1/4 cup hummus
Dinner: Cod and 1/4 cup mashed parsnips with side salad
Dessert: Fruit

MORE MEAL IDEAS

BREAKFAST

- Plain oatmeal, 1 cup berries, tea or coffee
- Egg-white omelet with mixed vegetables, tea or coffee
- Cheerios with skim milk, grapefruit, tea or coffee
- Nonfat Greek yogurt with almonds and berries, tea or coffee
- Nonfat ricotta with fruit
- High-protein cereal, berries, tea or coffee
- Pop Protein Shakes with milk or water and fruit

LUNCH

- Tuna salad made with low-fat or light mayonnaise and wrapped in lettuce
- Chicken or tuna salad over mixed green salad with oil and vinegar and an apple
- Chopped salad with sliced turkey and walnuts
- Spinach salad with crumbled farmer's blue cheese and an apricot
- Grilled chicken with green salad and an apple
- Shrimp cocktail with horseradish sauce or soy sauce with mixed green salad
- Sashimi with low-sodium soy sauce and green salad
- Romaine lettuce with vegetables and sunflower seeds
- Spinach salad with tomatoes and roasted chickpeas

DINNER

- Salmon, broccoli salad, blueberries
- Grilled chicken, mixed vegetables, strawberries
- Pan-seared tuna steaks, string beans, kiwi
- Lean flank steak, asparagus, salad
- Scallops sautéed with olive oil and spinach
- Pan-seared flounder, roasted peppers, raspberries
- Grilled chicken with low-fat cheddar cheese and green salad
- Tofu burger with green salad
- Eggplant casserole with salad and side of lentils
- Portobello mushroom topped with roasted tomatoes and hummus, with a green salad

SNACK

- Raw vegetables with hummus or guacamole
- Raw vegetables with tzatziki sauce (cucumber/dill sauce)
- Almonds with fruit
- Nonfat Greek yogurt with fruit or almonds
- Natural peanut butter or almond butter with sliced apple
- Turkey with low-fat cheese or avocado in lettuce wrap
- Low-fat string cheese with fruit or vegetables
- Low-fat cottage cheese with fruit
- Nonfat ricotta cheese with fruit or vegetables
- Nonfat ricotta cheese with dash of vanilla
- Tuna with vegetables
- Roasted chickpeas: drain chickpeas, put on pan, drizzle with olive oil, and bake 450 degrees for 40 to 50 minutes
- Celery with natural peanut butter or almond butter
- Pop snack bar

DESSERT

- Nonfat Greek yogurt with sliced apple and cinnamon
- Fresh fruit with nonfat Greek yogurt
- Baked apples with cinnamon

CHAPTER 24

DINING OUT

Unfortunately, quiet dinners at home every night have become the exception in most U.S. homes. Kids' activities and working long hours have made eating at restaurants and buzzing through drive-throughs a large part of our culture. While it's not optimal, I really believe that you can always find decent choices wherever you are. Here are some of our favorite Pop dining out tips.

First, try not to go out to dinner on an empty stomach or feeling starved. Eat as you normally would during the rest of the day, including snacks. Make dinner plans as early as possible so your eating schedule can remain consistent. Drink plenty of water during dinner and ask not to have bread put on your table before your meal. Ask how items are prepared and stay away from fried, breaded, crispy entrees and look for baked, broiled, steamed, or grilled foods instead. Avoid cream sauces and control what you eat by substituting a side of French fries, mashed potatoes, or rice for two vegetables or salad instead. Ask for all sauces and condiments on the side.

- Ask for your salad dressing on the side or use oil and vinegar instead.
- Eat slowly, allowing your body to feel satisfied so you avoid overeating.
- Have a sugar-free mint to end your meal.
- Consider wrapping a portion of your meal before you start eating.
- Do not feel you need to finish your meal if you are full; take note of your internal cues.

WHEN EATING AT AN ITALIAN RESTAURANT...

- Avoid foods containing words such as *alfredo*, *carbonara*, *saltimbocca*, *parmigiana*, *lasagna*, *manicotti*, and *stuffed*.
- Avoid foods that are fried, oily, or overly buttery.
- Avoid cream sauces, pestos, and meat sauces; instead, ask for a tomato-based sauce such as marinara.
- In dishes like eggplant Parmesan, ask for the eggplant to be baked instead of fried.
- Choose chicken or fish dishes that are grilled in vegetable-based or wine-based sauces.
- If you do order pasta, ask for whole-wheat or whole-grain pasta.

WHEN EATING AT A MEXICAN RESTAURANT...

- Avoid foods that are fried, such as chimichangas, nacho chips, and hard taco shells.
- Eat fajitas without the wrap.
- Ask for black beans and pinto beans instead of refried beans.

- Order chicken and seafood dishes rather than beef or pork dishes.
- Many Mexican dishes are covered in high-calorie cheese, sour cream, and guacamole; ask to have your meal served without those.
- Request salsa as a topping on the side.

WHEN EATING AT A CHINESE RESTAURANT...

- Avoid foods that are fried; instead, look for steamed foods.
- Try to avoid noodles, wontons, and egg rolls.
- Order steamed brown rice instead of fried rice or white rice.
- Request a low-sodium soy sauce instead of regular soy sauce.
- Choose dishes with vegetables that are stir-fried, grilled, or steamed.
- Avoid the tempura vegetables.
- Sweet and sour sauce, duck sauce, plum sauce, oyster sauce, and hoisin sauce are very sweet and should be avoided or asked to be placed on the side.

WHEN EATING AT A DELI...

- Choose lean meats like ham, turkey, or chicken rather than bologna, salami, or pepperoni.
- Choose whole-wheat or rye bread if you are having it on bread.
- Ask if they will wrap your meat in lettuce instead of bread.
- Avoid mayonnaise and oil on your sandwiches; instead, use mustard.

SMART CHOICES AT CHAIN RESTAURANTS

Always ask for a side of vegetables or salad to replace potatoes or rice, and always ask for salad dressings or sauces on the side.

APPLEBEE'S

Garlic Herb Salmon
Garlic Herb Chicken
Onion Soup Au Gratin
Steak and Portobello (without sauce)
Grilled Chili Lime Chicken Salad
Cajun Lime Tilapia (no corn salsa)

CHILI'S

Cup of Terlingua Chili (without sour cream/cheese) and a side salad

Chili's Classic Sirloin
Margarita Grilled Chicken
Guiltless Grilled Salmon
Guiltless Black Bean Burger (no bun)
Grilled Salmon with Garlic and Herbs
Southwest Cedar Plank Tilapia

HOULIHAN'S

Low Carb Burger
Low Carb Grilled Rosemary Chicken
Low Carb Coriander Grilled Salmon
Low Carb Grilled Shrimp Skewers

Fresh Fish Selection

Note: All low-carb meals are served with California Smashers (whipped cauliflower) instead of potatoes. Ask for no cheese and no bacon on the smashers.

OUTBACK STEAKHOUSE

Grilled Shrimp on the Barbie
Seared Ahi Tuna
House Salad (without croutons)
Grillers (without rice and pineapple)
All steaks
Outback Lamb (without sauce)
Chicken on the Barbie (without sauce)
All fish

P.F. CHANG'S

Hot & Sour Soup (cup)
Egg Drop Soup (cup)
Bikini Shrimp Salad
Buddha's Feast (steamed)
Garlic Snap Peas – Small
Spinach Stir-Fried with Garlic – Small

RED LOBSTER

Chilled Jumbo Shrimp Cocktail (with horseradish sauce, not cocktail sauce)

Live Maine Lobster
Garlic-Grilled Jumbo Shrimp
Snow Crab Legs
Tilapia (grilled or broiled)
Salmon (grilled or broiled)
Rainbow Trout (grilled or broiled)
Broiled Flounder
Grilled Chicken Breast
Garden Salad
Seasoned Broccoli

RUBY TUESDAY

Fresh Garden Bar
Grilled Chicken Salad
White Bean Chicken Chili
Grilled Salmon
Grilled Chicken
Petite Sirloin

T.G.I. FRIDAY'S

House Salad
Cobb Salad (without bacon)
Shrimp Key West
Petite Sirloin (replace side dish with vegetables)

THE CHEESECAKE FACTORY

Edamame
Weight Management Grilled Chicken

POP

Pan Seared Albacore Tuna
Tossed Green Salad
Boston House Salad (without bacon)
Herb Crusted Fillet of Salmon Salad
Seared Tuna Salad
Weight Management Pear & Endive Salad (without candied pecans)
Herb Crusted Fillet of Salmon
Wasabi Crusted Ahi Tuna
Petite Filet
Egg White Omelette
Energy Breakfast

CHAPTER 25

MAINTENANCE PHASE

Congratulations! You've made it to your goal weight, and now the trick is to maintain it. You now get to relax some of the rules from before, but you should still keep in mind these guidelines:

- Once you have achieved success during the weight reduction phase, slowly reintroduce grains and dairy back into your diet. The key will be portion control.
- Breads, pitas, pasta, rice, and wraps should be 100 percent whole wheat or 100 percent whole grain.
- Start with 1 slice of bread (consider a low-carb bread or wrap), 1/2 pita or wrap, or 1/2 cup of pasta or brown rice.
- Try to think of grains as condiments.
- Start adding more dairy (if desired and well tolerated by you) into your diet in moderation.
- Start adding vegetables and fruits with a higher glycemic index in small quantities, such as one small sweet potato, squash, carrots, beets, or a banana.

- Start adding back desserts in moderation, such as 1 ounce (3 to 4 small squares) of dark chocolate, at least 60 percent cocoa; fresh berries with a small amount of whipped cream; or low-sugar, low-carbohydrate ice cream or frozen yogurt (if full-fat ice cream, have just 1/5 cup).
- Allow yourself one glass of red or white wine.
- Ask at restaurants for healthier substitutions even if not on the menu (like fresh fruit for dessert).
- Ultimately, most people stay within five pounds of their goal weight. Be conscious of where you are with your weight, and if you see it trending upward, act immediately to correct the situation.

EPILOGUE

This book evolved from the many discussions we had about the thousands of people we had seen struggling with their weight. Although we had helped many, we were particularly focused on those whose progress was limited. Clearly those who made healthy food choices, incorporated exercise into their routines, and were able to adopt a new mind-set had the most success. Specifically, they realized their health and longevity depended on eating healthy foods and exercising. Those who succeeded had more energy and felt considerably better about themselves. Many who had failed previously were surprised but ecstatic about their progress and success. It was natural for them to have doubts at first when they had a history of failure, but they all learned that losing weight *can* be done — and in a healthy, long-term way.

We hope you have benefited from these stories and hearing about our patients' struggles with obesity and life's stresses. They were all determined to change and live the best life possible. If others can realize success, so can you.

Remember to send positive messages to yourself and avoid self-criticism. Focus on your strengths and strive to create a meaningful life. Become the person you want to be by always doing what makes you proud. With motivation and determination, you can be the person of your dreams. You have our best wishes for success.

—Dr. Rebecca Cipriano
—Dr. Kenneth Herman

ADDITIONAL RESOURCES

SAMPLE JOURNAL

Journaling is an important part of your weight loss journey. Here's a sample template for you to follow:

SAMPLE DAY

BREAKFAST

SNACK

LUNCH

SNACK

DINNER

TOTAL WEIGHT LOSS

DATE	WEIGHT	TOTAL WEIGHT LOSS

DATE: **WEEK:**

Breakfast

Snack

Lunch

Snack

Dinner

Today's feelings/questions/concerns:

Exercise

Water ☐☐☐☐☐☐☐☐☐☐☐☐☐☐☐☐☐☐☐☐☐

BODY MASS INDEX CHART

BMI	19	20	21	22	23	24	25	26	27	28	29	30	35	40
Height	Weight (in pounds)													
4'10"	91	96	100	105	110	115	119	124	129	134	138	143	167	191
4'11"	94	99	104	109	114	119	124	128	133	138	143	148	173	198
5'0"	97	102	107	112	118	123	128	133	138	143	148	153	179	204
5'1"	100	106	111	116	122	127	132	137	143	148	153	158	185	211
5'2"	104	109	115	120	126	131	136	142	147	153	158	164	191	218
5'3"	107	113	118	124	130	135	141	146	152	158	163	169	197	225
5'4"	110	116	122	128	134	140	145	151	157	163	169	174	204	232
5'5"	114	120	126	132	138	144	150	156	162	168	174	180	210	240
5'6"	118	124	130	136	142	148	155	161	167	173	179	186	216	247
5'7"	121	127	134	140	146	153	159	166	172	178	185	191	223	255
5'8"	125	131	138	144	151	158	164	171	177	184	190	197	230	262
5'9"	128	135	142	149	155	162	169	176	182	189	196	203	236	270
5'10"	132	139	146	153	160	167	174	181	188	195	202	207	243	278
5'11"	136	143	150	157	165	172	179	186	193	200	208	215	250	286
6'0"	140	147	154	162	169	177	184	191	199	206	213	221	258	294
6'1"	144	151	159	166	174	182	189	197	204	212	219	227	265	302
6'2"	148	155	163	171	179	186	194	202	210	218	225	233	272	311
6'3"	152	160	168	176	184	192	200	208	216	224	232	240	279	319
6'4"	156	164	172	180	189	197	205	213	221	230	238	246	287	328

Source: www.bmi-calculator.net/bmi-chart.php

EXERCISE GUIDELINES

- You must exercise a minimum of 30 minutes a day. Work up to it if you have to. The daily habit is the most important part.

- If you are not breaking a sweat, you are not working hard enough.
- People who exercise while making changes to their diet lose more weight. Research shows that people who lose more than 30 pounds and keep it off more than a year walk an average of four miles a day.
- Exercise will help reduce the stress in your life. Find the exercises that work for you and a daily time that you can stick with.
- Cardio workouts can be fast walking, running, biking, or dancing (see calorie-burning chart on the next page). Exercises like jumping jacks, sit-ups, and push-ups are very effective.
- Pilates and yoga are abdominal-based workouts that are ideal for postpartum, perimenopausal, and menopausal women. Toning and strength training are reserved for when you are closer to your goal.
- We cannot stress the importance of exercise enough. It is impossible to lose weight and keep it off if you do not have a great diet, exercise, and behavioral modification.

CALORIES BURNED

Activity (1-hour duration)	and calories burned		
	160 pounds	200 pounds	240 pounds
Aerobics, high impact	533	664	796
Aerobics, low impact	365	455	545
Aerobics, water	402	501	600
Backpacking	511	637	763
Basketball game	584	728	872
Bicycling, < 10 mph, leisure	292	364	436
Bowling	219	273	327
Canoeing	256	319	382
Dancing, ballroom	219	273	327

Football, touch or flag	584	728	872
Golfing, carrying clubs	314	391	469
Hiking	438	546	654
Ice skating	511	637	763
Racquetball	511	637	763
Resistance (weight) training	365	455	545
Rollerblading	548	683	818
Rope jumping	861	1,074	1,286
Rowing, stationary	438	546	654
Running, 5 mph	606	755	905
Running, 8 mph	861	1,074	1,286
Skiing, cross-country	496	619	741
Skiing, downhill	314	391	469
Skiing, water	438	546	654
Softball or baseball	365	455	545
Stair treadmill	657	819	981
Swimming, laps	423	528	632
Tae kwon do	752	937	1,123
Tai chi	219	273	327
Tennis, singles	584	728	872
Volleyball	292	364	436
Walking, 2 mph	204	255	305
Walking, 3.5 mph	314	391	469

Source: www.mayoclinic.com/health/exercie/SM00109

IMMUNITY FOOD LIST

Anti-Cancer/Anti-Infection Foods
arugula
bok choy
broccoli and broccoli rabe

Brussels sprouts
cabbage
cauliflower
collard greens
horseradish
kale
kohlrabi
mustard greens
radishes
red cabbage
turnip greens
watercress

Anti-Inflammatory/Anti-Tumor/Anti–Fat Cell Foods

berries
chives
cinnamon
citrus fruits
flaxseeds
garlic
ginger
grapes
green tea
leeks
mushrooms
omega-3 fats
onions
peppers
pomegranates
scallions
shallots

soybeans
spinach
tomatoes
turmeric

Top 10 Immunity Foods
arugula
berries
broccoli
Brussels sprouts
cabbage
collards
garlic
kale
lettuce (green)
mushrooms
mustard greens
onions
pomegranates
seeds (flax, chia, sesame, sunflower)
tomatoes
watercress

ABOUT THE AUTHORS

Dr. Rebecca Cipriano is a well-respected and in-demand medical doctor, board-certified in obstetrics and gynecology, who's been in private practice for more than 15 years. Known for her warmth, candor, and professionalism, she is the co-founder of Healthy Woman OB/GYN, one of the most popular OB/GYN groups in New Jersey. After years of caring for women of all ages and walks of life, she recognized the rapidly emerging need for nutrition counseling as a means of prevention as well as panacea for what ails them.

Governed by the breadth of knowledge she obtained via her master's degree in clinical nutrition and guided by her passion to help patients live a healthy life on all levels, she founded A Better You Weight Management Centers in 2008. More than a typical weight loss program, A Better You offered medically supervised, one-on-one nutrition counseling with a goal of teaching people how to not just lose the weight but keep it off for life. Dr. Rebecca is a pioneer in the field of personalized weight loss and advocates for health and fitness as a nonnegotiable lifestyle change, rather than a trend or quick fix.

As A Better You bloomed, so did Dr. Rebecca's media profile, including speaking engagements and televised appearances with wellness luminaries like Deepak Chopra and Dr. Oz, which positioned her as a top expert on medically supervised weight loss and nutrition as a lifestyle choice.

Ever fueled by her desire to educate and empower men, women, and children on the real way to lose weight and feel better, Dr. Rebecca began putting pen to paper in 2011 to create this book. In early 2012, she also set the wheels in motion to elevate the allure of her already booming weight loss business (which at the time of this printing has helped thousands of people lose a combined total weight of more than 37,000 pounds) by rebranding it as Pop Weight Loss, a nationally franchised program that delivers her tried-and-true personalized weight loss solutions to everyone.

Dr. Rebecca believes that proper nutrition, as supported by regular exercise and a set schedule, is the catalyst for all positive change in your life. Her program calls on a mind-body connection that activates each person to effect real and lasting change that nourishes a life in which excess weight (and the health problems it causes) are no longer an issue.

Dr. Kenneth Herman is a board-certified clinical psychologist and a fellow in the American Academy of Clinical Psychology. He was the founder and director of the Psychological Service Center in Teaneck, N.J., for many years. Throughout his 50-year career in the field of mental health as a psychotherapist, he has also taught on the university level, lectured extensively, conducted research, and appeared on multiple radio and television programs. Dr. Herman is the author of *Secrets from the Sofa: A Psychologist's Guide to Achieving Personal Peace*. Readers' comments and reviews may be seen on his website at www.secretsfromthesofa. com.

Secrets from the Sofa was a USA Book News Finalist in the categories of College Guide and Health: Psychology/ Mental Health, and first runner-up in the Eric Hoffer Award in the category of Health, among other awards. The content of the manuscript is based on cognitive/behavioral psychology and Dr. Herman's experience and research. Dr. Herman presents the tools and skills that he has found effective in interacting with thousands of patients. He shares how people can correct the negative thoughts, perceptions, and habits that stand in the way of achieving one's goals. With encouragement and support, he guides readers to be strong emotionally and cope effectively with life's stresses. He presents case studies to show how many of his patients have changed. His message to people who want to lose weight, eat healthy, and stay in shape is this: It is possible to change. Many others have persevered and achieved their goals. You can, too.

Dr. Herman feels that he and Dr. Rebecca have taken the mystery out of how to eat well and stay physically fit. He appeals to readers to follow their lead and be selective regarding their food choices and realize that they are being presented with lifetime suggestions that will stave off illness and be personally rewarding. He believes the content of this book is the ammunition for the change and good feelings individuals are seeking.

ACKNOWLEDGMENTS

My father and I would like to thank our editor, Haley Shapley, for her hard work in organizing and editing our material. You brought our work into a cohesive form and we very much appreciate your dedication to the project.

Thank you to Lisbeth Harding for inspiring graphic design work that brings our words to life and makes them *pop*.

I would also like to thank Stephanie Leonetti, the director of my weight loss program, for her help with research and editing of this book and her mission to make good nutrition an everyday event. I also credit Stephanie with her persistence in helping me open my first center, and I appreciate her shared passion in helping people achieve goals they did not think were possible.

I thank my husband and life partner for pushing me to pursue my passion and teaching me to dream big.

To Jillian Swartz-Hoagland, I am grateful for your help with writing ideas and giving structure initially to this manuscript. Thank you for always being available to be a sounding board for the book and for your ever-creative ideas.

Thanks to the photographers of the author photos, taken by Gary Gellman (Dr. Cipriano) and Ron Aubert (Dr. Herman).

Last but not least, I am grateful to my patients, who have taught me that it is never too late to change your life for the better. Congratulations on all that you have achieved.